The Secondary SLP Roadmap

PRAISE FOR *THE SECONDARY SLP ROADMAP*

"SLPs working with older students finally have a go-to guide that was actually written with this population in mind. Hallie's roadmap is full of time-saving strategies, helpful frameworks, and real-life wisdom—whether you're a new grad or have been in the field for years, it's a resource you'll come back to again and again."
— **Dr. Angelyn Franks**, Burnout Coach and SLP

"Hallie's passion for the field of speech-language pathology has always been evident, and her commitment to supporting both students and fellow professionals continues to inspire. In *The Secondary SLP Roadmap*, she brings a much-needed resource to the often overlooked realm of secondary education, offering clear strategies, practical tools, and a supportive voice that speaks directly to the challenges SLPs face when working with older students.

Her experience, insight, and innovative approaches make this book not only an essential guide for new clinicians, but also a refreshing reference for seasoned professionals looking to make a greater impact at the middle and high school levels.

Hallie's work reflects the same dedication and thoughtfulness she demonstrated as a student, and *The Secondary SLP Roadmap* is a testament to her continued growth and leadership in our field. I wholeheartedly recommend this book to any SLP looking to navigate the complexities of secondary education with clarity and confidence."
— **Matthew Kostel**, Special Education and Consultation Administrator

"Not too sure about schools? Hallie Sherman's *The Secondary SLP Roadmap* is the ideal place to begin. With clarity and compassion, she eases your mind, addresses your concerns, and provides real-world solutions that will guide you through your best school year yet. This book is the perfect complement to graduate coursework, an absolute must-have for clinical fellows, and a supportive sidekick for experienced clinicians alike. Say YES to this roadmap and get ready for an amazing adventure—perfect for elementary SLPs, too!"
— **Elsha Young**, MS, CCC-SLP

"Inspiring and practical, this book is a must-have for school-based speech-language pathologists. With clarity and compassion, it offers invaluable tools for navigating conversations with administrators, teachers, and parents alike. Rich with clinical writing guidance and intervention strategies tailored for older students, it's an engaging resource that bridges real-world challenges with effective, actionable solutions."
— **Dr. Melissa P. Garcia**, CCC-SLP

The Secondary SLP Roadmap

Motivating Students to Crush Their Speech and Language Goals

HALLIE SHERMAN

JB JOSSEY-BASS™

A Wiley Brand

Published by John Wiley & Sons, Inc., Hoboken, New Jersey.
Published simultaneously in Canada.

ISBNs: 9781394301713 (Paperback), 9781394301751 (ePDF), 9781394301737 (epub)

Library of Congress Control Number: 2025041096 **(print)**

Cover Design: Wiley
Author Photo: © Jennifer Lam

Printed and bound by CPI Group (UK) Ltd, Croydon, CR0 4YY

C9781394301713_240925

Contents

Visit https://speechtimefun.com/book to access free resources for this book.

Acknowledgments   ix

About the Author   xi

Preface   xiii

Introduction   xvii

SECTION 1
Getting Quick Wins   1

CHAPTER 1
Start Small, Win Big   3

CHAPTER 2
The Role of the SLP with Secondary Students   9

CHAPTER 3
Determining Where to Start with Older Speech Students   23

CHAPTER 4
Teaching Strategies and Techniques   43

CHAPTER 5
Connection over Data Collection   63

SECTION 2

   Creative Competence   **73**

CHAPTER 6
   The Importance of Incorporating Student Interests and Goals   **75**

CHAPTER 7
   Building Rapport   **87**

CHAPTER 8
   Routines and Expectations   **99**

SECTION 3

   The 60-Minute Plan Strategy   **109**

CHAPTER 9
   A Plan for Work-Life Balance   **111**

CHAPTER 10
   Feeling Relevant Without Using the Curriculum   **123**

CHAPTER 11
   Adapting Resources and Using Fewer Materials   **135**

CHAPTER 12
   Mixed Groups Made Easy   **147**

CHAPTER 13
   Building Articulation and Social Skills   **159**

CHAPTER 14
   What About Life Skills?   **169**

Conclusion   **191**

Index   **195**

Acknowledgments

This book would not have been possible without a few special people in my life who support me unconditionally. To my supportive husband, Geoff. Thank you for being patient with me and for always being my biggest cheerleader. You have been by my side since undergrad when I decided to start my education to be an SLP. Love you and the life we have created together. To my daughters, Ella and Addison. I hope to show you that anything is possible if you work hard and put your mind to it. Reach for the stars. Mommy loves you and sorry for always working. To my parents, thank you for teaching me about hard work and dedication and maybe also teaching me about this field. Thank you for providing babysitting and support. Thank you also to all of my mentors and business coaches throughout the years. You have shown me what is possible and helped me go for my dreams.

To all of the SLPs who have purchased my resources and products throughout the years, you push me each and every day to be the best SLP and CEO. I wouldn't be here if it weren't for you. Keep making an impact each and every day with your students.

About the Author

Hallie Sherman, M.S. CCC-SLP, is a licensed speech-language pathologist in New York. She worked in public schools for over 15 years before she left to work as the CEO full time for Speech Time Fun, Inc. At Speech Time Fun, Inc., Hallie provides materials and trainings for SLPs working with grades 4–12 to help them plan with ease and confidence. She does this through her SLP Elevate membership, her TPT resources, her podcast SLP Coffee Talk, her virtual conference she hosts three times a year called the Speech Retreat, and other various trainings for organizations and associations. Visit https://speechtimefun.com to learn more about Hallie and her work.

Preface

Dear Reader,

It means the world to me that you have decided to read this book. I am Hallie Sherman, and I am a licensed speech-language pathologist (SLP) in New York. I also hold the Teacher of Students with Speech and Language Disabilities (TSSLD) certification. I graduated from the University of Buffalo with a degree in communication sciences and disorders. I went into undergraduate studies completely undecided about my major. I knew I wanted to work with children and make a difference, but I did not want to become a teacher. I found out about the SLP field from a friend taking some classes, and I tried one out and fell in love with it. I was never an amazing student, but I found it easy to study and ended up graduating with honors.

I continued my path to become an SLP at Adelphi University, where I graduated with my master's degree in speech-language pathology. I knew I was destined to work in a school setting. I loved having the ability to collaborate with other educators, and I even enjoyed working with groups and preferred it over individual therapy. I realized I enjoyed working with school-aged children and this was where I was meant to be.

When you love what you do, you love to talk about it and help others along the way. I love helping SLPs be the best they can be. It has been a labor of love to write this book, and I cannot wait to see how many SLPs, SLPAs, CFs, and graduate students it can help and inspire. I always wished there was a guide or a curriculum to show me exactly what to do with my older students. I hope this book can be that guide that will show you exactly what to do, what not to do, and prevent you from making the mistakes that I made when trying to adapt lessons meant for children under the age of 10 to upper elementary, middle, and high schoolers.

I would have never guessed I would be writing a book like this when I started my career as an SLP. As a brand-new graduate, full of possibility, I started my career working with preschoolers. I realized right away that age group was not for me. I always knew I wanted to work with school-aged students, but with the job market at the time I had to take whatever I could. I went on what it felt like a million job interviews. On one of my toughest days in the preschool, I left early for an interview for a split position in a middle and high school. I was shocked to find out that I was asked to return the next day for a demonstration lesson. Of course, I only had one business suit at the time so I had to run to buy a second outfit for the next day and had to figure out what in the world I would do with those students. I had never worked with older students. I had done my graduate school placement with elementary students. I decided to call my friend who was working in a middle school at the time. She reminded me that middle schoolers are just big kids, and they have similar needs as the elementary students. Just use their interests, she told me, and you will be good to go. I prepared an entire recalling directions activity with a baseball theme. I got the job. I couldn't believe it.

That was the start of my school-based career. But unfortunately, it was only a leave replacement. I hopped from leave replacement to leave replacement until I finally landed a tenure track position in a district, where I filled a leave replacement for two years working with fifth and sixth graders. Once again, I found myself working with older students. I had to learn again what my role was, how to motivate them, and how to make my lessons effective.

I made a lot of mistakes in the early years of my career. I did not want anyone to realize I was unsure of myself or lacked confidence. I was afraid to ask for help. I was also the only SLP in my building, and I had a caseload that was growing larger and larger each year. I was also working in sweltering hot classrooms, dealing with fertility issues, and trying to just build connections with my colleagues who did not understand my struggles. Did I mention that I am only five feet tall and my students were taller than me?

You will hear a lot about my specific mistakes in various areas throughout this book. But once I figured out what worked with my students and how to get them from bored to onboard, I knew I had to share it with the world. I started my blog, Speech Time Fun, in 2012. I thought it would be just an online journal to share what was working with my students. It was more for therapeutic purposes. I did not expect anyone to find it, let alone read it. However, there was apparently a need for ideas and support for SLPs working with older students, and SLPs everywhere were finding my blog posts and sharing them on Pinterest. They were asking me to write more and asking me for more help. In August 2012, I opened my Teachers Pay Teachers store and posted my first resource. It was "Cause and Effect Cupcakes." It sold instantly after I posted it, and I realized SLPs needed more for older students. There wasn't a curriculum or a place to purchase motivating resources for this age group. I kept creating, writing passages, and adding more resources that were unique for this age group.

I knew I wanted to help more and wanted to share more than just resources. I wanted to share how to motivate older students, how to plan quickly, and how to keep the fun in speech therapy. I started presenting for several online conferences, state and local associations, and even presented at the 2016 ASHA Convention. I loved being able to provide SLPs with relevant and practical professional development that left them feeling like they had what they needed to get the job done the very next day. That was when I created the Speech Retreat conference that has helped inspire and motivate SLPs around the world and bring speakers that are able to share top trends in the field and innovative practices that school-based SLPs can use immediately.

I decided to take my passion for professional development and my love of creating motivating resources for grades 4–12 and started my SLP Elevate membership in 2021, a program where I offer materials, training, and support for SLPs working with grades 4–12 (learn more at slpelevate.com). I wanted a space where like-minded and passionate SLPs could get unlimited access to resources that were appropriate for older students yet simplified so they could be successful with them. I wanted to be able to provide training and support that does not exist anywhere else for working with this age group. I have helped thousands of SLPs and their students see tons of success and have more fun. I resigned from my district position in June 2023 so that I could focus my energy on Speech Time Fun, Inc., and be able to provide more support through my various offerings and platforms. I absolutely love being a speech-language pathologist and love that I now get to teach and coach SLPs so that they continue to love what they do and have more of a work-life balance.

My mission is to help inspire and empower speech-language pathologists working with grades 4–12 by providing them with the tools, understanding, and resources necessary so that they can help their students succeed. More importantly, the more fun you have each day, the more fun your students will have in return. As a mom of two young daughters, at the time of writing this book they are 10 and 6 years old, I know what it is like to have a busy life outside of work and want to be as present as possible. I am determined to help all SLPs leave more work at work and be able to spend more time with the ones they love outside of work. You can still love what you do and make a difference while putting yourself and your loved ones first.

I am excited to share with you the frameworks that I have established for working with this age group in this book. It is the resource I wish I had when I started. I am so excited to hear about your wins after reading this book. I hope you share your lightbulb moments with me.

XOXO,
Hallie

Introduction

This book is a unique resource for speech-language pathologists because there isn't much out there for those working with secondary students. Although this book is a guide, it is also filled with stories and practical ideas that you can use right away. You will walk away with tangible tips and tricks that I have used with my own students and that have been used by those that I have supported over the years through my professional development trainings and my SLP Elevate membership (my program where I offer materials, training, and support for SLPs working with grades 4–12; learn more at `slpelevate.com`).

SLPs often struggle to know how to effectively work with secondary students. Students in kindergarten through third grade are easier to motivate and are often not yet aware of their difficulties. Once they hit the fourth grade and they are reading to learn, they are more aware that learning is difficult for them. This book contains three phases that SLPs can go through. It includes frameworks to know where to start, how to determine goals, how to teach skills differently, how to engage students, and how to adapt resources to meet all the needs of their students. By utilizing all the frameworks and going through the three phases, SLPs can confidently work with secondary students and see massive progress.

This book is for you if you are new to working with secondary students, struggling to get students motivated, having a hard time determining goals, or spending way too much time planning for your sessions. As SLPs, we are always learning and growing. This book is another way for you to learn new techniques to improve your practice and have an impact with your students. I share stories about my career, mistakes I made, lessons my own students taught me, and more.

You have two choices—you can keep reading to learn about my experiences and what has worked with my students and the SLPs I have helped over the years, or you can close this book, not try something new, and continue to wonder how to motivate these older students. You may continue to feel ineffective. You may even consider trying to find a new setting or age group to work with. It may not be easy, but it can be so rewarding when you find what works and see the spark in a young adolescent.

HOW TO USE THIS BOOK

Each of the three phases makes up a section of this book. Each phase has three components. Even if you feel like you have a handle on one of the phases or aspects within a phase, I suggest you still read the section or chapter. Once you have a deeper understanding of each phase, you can execute a lesson with confidence and plan in less than one hour a week. Go through the phases in order. They were designed to build upon each other.

As you move through the book, you will learn how to set yourself up for success, how to engage your students, and how to use your resources effectively to keep preparation time to a minimum. Imagine being able to walk into any session feeling prepared and confident. Imagine being able to have the energy to focus on the students in front of you.

I also put together supplemental resources for you that you can access on my website, at www.speechtimefun.com/book. I will reference many resources throughout this book. You can gather them all at this one link. We learn best by doing, so you can access lots of tools and resources to help you utilize the frameworks discussed in this book. My goal is that you can use what you learn right away and have quick wins with your students. It builds confidence and helps with momentum to learn more. I cannot wait for you to learn all about these resources and get the opportunity to use them with your students.

WHO IS THIS BOOK FOR?

After working with thousands of SLPs, I recognize the need for more training and support when it comes to working with this age group. I did not learn these techniques in graduate school. I had to learn them on my own and make a ton of mistakes. Over the years, I have also worked with many graduate students as their supervisor of their school practicum, and they have lacked prior knowledge on how to work with this age group.

This book is for graduate students looking to learn as much as they can while they are in school. This can be part of a book study, graduate curriculum, or a way to prepare for an upcoming placement with this age group. This book is also for new SLPs or SLPs who are newly hired to work with secondary students. This book is also for veteran SLPs who have been working with older students for years and want to refine their skills and see even bigger results. This book is for any SLP working with self-contained students, life skills students, students in a general education setting, providing push-in services, or providing pull-out services.

You can even use the concepts in this book if you are working via teletherapy. No matter what your situation, if you work with grades 4–12, you will get value out of this book.

No matter where you are on your career or education path, you can benefit from learning from my experiences. We are often alone on our SLP island and can benefit from learning from others with similar experiences. We all want the best for our students, and we are also lifelong learners. There is a need for more training and resources for older students, and that is why I have written this book for you.

WHAT THIS BOOK IS NOT

If you are just looking for pages and pages of theory and research, this book is not for you. If you are looking for a boring read to help you sleep at night, this book is not for you. This isn't a textbook. It is a practical guide, with stories, strategies, and fun ideas you can use right away. I won't be going into thorough details about specific disorders, AAC (augmentive and alternative communication), or other specific topics. I share overall concepts that can be applied to all goals and situations. I also share what has worked for me and the many SLPs I have worked with over the years.

MY WHY

I am writing this book because I have seen such a huge need for more education and collaboration with SLPs working with upper grades. Unless you did a graduate program placement with this age group, you probably never received formal education in working with this age group. We are also often the only ones in our buildings or districts working with this age group and can feel alone. I hear so many stories of SLPs on the brink of burnout or too overwhelmed to consider staying in the school system. That breaks my heart because there are so many students who need our help and can benefit from prepared and confident SLPs to take on this age group.

I often see SLPs in Facebook groups asking about working with this age group. They are either asking if they should consider the change or when they have started with this age group and feel completely lost and overwhelmed. Our students in this age group need us and we can make such an impact. We just need the confidence to go into each and every day to show up and be our best. I am here to help make that possible.

I fully believe that everything happens for a reason. I was meant to land a job with this age group, was meant to make mistakes, and was meant to figure things out so that I could be your guide. In fact, the day of my interview for a position in a middle and high school I actually got peed on by a preschooler! It was my clinical fellowship year, and I put my résumé out to school districts just to see what was out there and my options. I ran home, showered 10 times, and went into that interview ready to work with a different age group. I got that job. Clearly, it was meant to be.

If you know someone who can benefit from motivation, or if you know of a new graduate that just got hired to work with this age group, share the love and let them know about this book. The more resources there are to help, the better we can all be together. This field is amazing. We went into it to make a difference. It shouldn't matter the setting or the age group. We can all have the necessary training and tools to get the job done and make a huge impact.

NOW WHAT?

After each chapter, I challenge you to try something new and be open to a new perspective. Just like we want our students to experience wins and build confidence, my hope is that you do too. So, before you go on to the next chapter, I want you to think about your "why" and jot it down on a sticky note or somewhere for you to reflect on. Why did you become an SLP? Why did you decide to work in a school or in the setting you are in? Why did you decide to work with secondary students? Your answer may be that you were forced or it's just where the job placed you. That is okay. Jot it down. Your why will always ground you and remind you to keep going when things get tough. Every day won't be rainbows and unicorns when working in this field, especially working with challenging teenagers. But you are making a difference, and your students are so lucky to have you.

If you are ready to learn more about what to work on with your current or future speech students grades 4–12, let's dive into the first section. Let's start making magic and have a massive impact.

Getting Quick Wins

In this section, which includes Chapters 1 through 5, you'll learn about the benefits of and how to achieve quick wins with your students. This isn't about making things too easy for them, but about presenting concepts at the appropriate level for them so that they can see what is possible. We want them to realize they can overcome challenges, do hard things, and see success. If we want them willing to work with us as things get harder and even more challenging, we have to start somewhere. We must get them a quick win and build momentum. If you are struggling to know exactly what goals to address, how to teach skills so that students' grasp them, and how to feel confident in your role as an SLP working with this age group, this section can help!

CHAPTER 1

Start Small, Win Big

I will never forget when I started working with upper grades. I did not do my school placement with this age, I did not learn how to work with this age group in graduate school, and I did not know anyone working with this age group I could ask questions. This was a time before social media, before iPhones, before Pinterest, and before Teachers Pay Teachers. I was terrified. It did not help that I did not want to work with this age group. I wanted to work with elementary students. But a job was a job and I was not going to pass an opportunity up. I did not want anyone suspecting I was not capable.

On top of not having experience or materials, I had an extremely large caseload. I stopped counting after 60 students. A large caseload, a large building with lots of personalities to adjust to, and lots of different goals to manage. Back-to-back sessions, large groups of five students, students all working on different goals, and trying to navigate a new setting. It was a huge adjustment. To add to the stress of all this, I was placed in a tiny room that was hot. There was zero circulation of air. No windows. Just heat pumping in and nowhere to go. I was even forced to keep the door closed for security reasons. Enough said.

Okay. Back to the caseload. I was given Individualized Education Plans (IEPs) with goals such as determining the main idea, making inferences, recalling sequences, and understanding vocabulary. I did not even realize those were things students in grades 4–12 would still be working on or need to be working on in speech therapy. Yes, when I did my school placement with elementary students, we had some sequencing and basic answering questions goals (i.e., who, what, where, when, why) but not as complex as these. I learned how to work on more basic skills, even using literacy-based therapy, but I was never instructed how to work on these goals.

I remember seeing similar goals listed to be addressed by the classroom teacher and wondered why we were both working on them. I knew why reading specialists would be working on reading goals. But why me too? Should we both be working on that? What was my role with these goals and why was it a speech thing?

I did not have any resources to look at. I walked into an empty therapy room. I only had the materials I made and collected from my elementary placement. What should I be using to work on these goals? I also didn't have any colleagues to ask questions. I was the only SLP in the building. So, I did what I had to do; I went into the local teacher store that existed at the time. I found English language arts (ELA) workbooks from various publishers. The store employee could not help me find speech therapy materials, but they directed me to what they had for the above goals. I found ESL worksheets from free websites. I used what I had and went through the motions. I assumed this was what I was expected and supposed to be doing and using with my students. I didn't see other options. After a few weird comments from students, I learned to use whiteout to cover up the ESL label on the worksheets.

Worksheet after worksheet. We just practiced the various goals over and over again. I remember thinking, I guess this is what I am supposed to do and what I am supposed to use to work on these goals. I didn't have anyone telling me otherwise. It also didn't help that I was new, no one knew who I was, and I was having a difficult time getting teachers to let me know how my students were doing in the classroom or what they were working on. I didn't have access to the curriculum, textbooks, or what things they were trying in the classroom. At the time, many of the classroom teachers I was working with wouldn't even respond to an email I sent. I left notes in their mailboxes, and they did not respond.

It did work for a while. My students participated and did the work. Were they making progress toward their IEP goals? Were they becoming a more effective communicator or student? I am not sure. Were they having fun? Probably not. But they did the work, and I was getting the job done. I was addressing the goals as defined on their IEPs. But I did not feel adequate or effective, and major imposter syndrome was kicking in. Who was I to be working on these skills with these students? I did not feel properly trained or prepared. I was still a relatively new clinician, and working with this age group was foreign to me. I was not seeing quick wins, let alone any wins. I was not seeing progress at all, and I felt like I wasn't making an impact.

INTRODUCING MY MOST CHALLENGING STUDENT EVER

But then I had a student who I'll call K. Have you ever had that one student that you will never forget, but not for positive reasons? K. did not like my activities. He did not like me. He did not have a problem letting me and the other students know how he felt. He would torment me and the other students every time he entered my speech room. He complained about every activity. "This is boring." "This is babyish." "X is stupid for being here." He made me brace for impact and take a deep breath every time he was about to show up. (And of course he was never absent! Those students never are!). Week after week went on like this. It got worse over time. My anxiety when he entered the room grew. I was not confident. I was nervous, and it probably showed. I spent hours planning for his group because I did not want to have another disaster session that left me wanting to run out of the room and cry in the bathroom (no time to run to the car!). I knew I couldn't go the entire year stressing and worrying about planning for this one student on my caseload. I had 60 other students to worry about. I realized I had to ask for help and that I wasn't the only one working with this student. I asked his teachers, reading specialist, and even his former speech-language pathologist about him. "How is he doing in your class?" "How is his behavior?" "How are you getting him to partici-pate?" "Why is he receiving speech services?"

By asking the right questions, I finally found the answers I needed. I realized why he was acting the way he was and why he was receiving speech in the first place. K. couldn't read. He was in the sixth grade and reading on a kindergarten level. No wonder he was acting the way he was in my room. I was giving him reading comprehension activities, worksheets with passages he couldn't read. He did not want his peers to know he couldn't read. He was using his behavior as an avoidance strategy and boy was it working. But how could I work on the reading comprehension goals he had without reading?

I realized I needed a different approach. Did I have to make him read? What did he truly need from me? I started to understand my role as the SLP and with language comprehension and how I could support him without even reading. I started using a strengths-based approach and built his strengths to support his weaknesses. He was savvy socially, had strong listening comprehension skills, and had great background knowledge. I used materials that were appropriate for him. I did not force him to read. I used simplified language activities that he had background knowledge of. He was competitive and liked to win, so I incorporated games and competitions.

We played jeopardy games where I gave the students the option to read or to have me read to them. I found articles on his favorite sports but did not require him to read. I rewrote articles I found so that it was simplified and easier to understand. We solved mysteries where students worked together to figure out the mystery. I started using YouTube videos to work on comprehension skills.

I helped him achieve some quick wins and in so doing, built his confidence. He was willing to work for me and ended up becoming one of my star students. He learned my room was safe and he was capable there. I didn't provide him with activities that were so easy that he felt they were babyish or so challenging that he needed to avoid them. I changed the way I taught the skills so that he could grasp them and make tons of progress. I ended up discharging him from speech services on his IEP at the end of sixth grade.

By learning how to work with my most challenging student of my career thus far (and probably the most challenging throughout the years), I realized what was necessary to get quick wins for my students and how essential those wins were. We cannot just work on the end goal from the beginning and expect our students to be successful. We need to start where they are at and build up from there.

READY FOR QUICK WINS?

That is how I came up with the Quick Wins Concept. It is what I have used to guide me to knowing what to work on and how to work on it with my students. I didn't have a roadmap or curriculum, so I needed to develop something to provide me with direction. I have realized the importance of getting quick wins for students. I have also seen the frustration when they are not making progress or not understanding what we are doing. I cannot predict every situation for you. But I can help you determine what is appropriate for your individual students on your caseload. Yes, there are exceptions to every rule. Of course. But SLPs are creative problem solvers and use their knowledge and expertise for those situations. There are many components that will be necessary in order to achieve quick wins that we will go into thoroughly throughout this section. My goal is that you see the benefit of getting quick wins for your students and how to get them.

Some questions to think about:

- Do you find it challenging to come up with goals for your students?
- Do you struggle to know whether or not a student qualifies for speech?
- Do you have students that are not making the progress you would like?
- Do you find it challenging to work on goals so students they grasp them?

- Do you often find yourself feeling like a tutor or reading teacher?
- Does it take a long time to write evaluation reports or IEPs?
- Do you have a bunch of students on your caseload that you feel like should be dismissed or have nothing to work on anymore?

If you said "yes" to any of these questions, this section is for you. Even if you said "no" to any of these questions, don't skip this section of the book, since it gives you the foundation for the following sections, where I explain ways to motivate your students and plan quickly. But that isn't possible if you don't have a deep understanding of what to work on and how to work on it. You may even get a new nugget of information that will transform the way you view working with this age group. This section takes you through how to make these decisions and gives you the steps to take so you can write IEPs and teach the skills so your students grasp them and make progress. I have been there. I made many mistakes, as you read above. My hope is to help others get results faster and easier than I did.

In this section, I show you how you can get quick wins for your students. I go through in more detail how to determine where your students are, your role as an SLP in language comprehension and overall reading success, how to determine appropriate and attainable goals that can be met, and how to teach skills differently so that students can grasp them. We want to show our students they can be successful and build that momentum so that when things get more challenging as the year goes on, they won't give up, and they continue to push through. In addition, although every student can benefit from support, it is important for SLPs to truly understand who really warrants their services. This will help make appropriate recommendations and not have students on caseloads who are better suited to stay in the classroom.

If you find that your students are often not mastering goals or you are unsure how to teach the skills in a way that is different from the classroom teacher, take notes in this section. Imagine this: You have a new student to assess. You know exactly what to look for, what to determine, and how to generate goals and a game plan that will make a difference for that student. This is all possible with this Quick Wins Blueprint. Gone are the days of making arbitrary decisions and seeing arbitrary results.

My hope is that after reading this section, you feel equipped to make appropriate recommendations, create goals, and have a game plan on how to target those goals. We want our students crushing their goals and no longer needing us. We want to feel effective and that we are making an impact on our students and providing value when we take them out of the classroom. By making sure our goals and plan are tailored to the specific and individual needs of our students, we can ensure they are going to get the support they need to make progress with us that will carry over into the classroom.

How confident are you with the goals that your students have? Do you believe they are the best goals to meet their needs? Do you feel confident in knowing how to address these goals? Take a moment to reflect on that. Then, head onto the next chapter and learn how to better understand your role with this age group. This section will help you determine which goals to work on and how to answer the question "Why do I have to go to speech?!"

CHAPTER 2

The Role of the SLP with Secondary Students

When I started working with secondary students, I was shocked to see that they still received speech therapy. I had students with various levels of capabilities and in different classroom settings. The majority of my students were in self-contained or collaborative classrooms. Therefore, they were also receiving special education services. I was not the only one working with them. Many were also receiving reading support from a reading specialist. I was pulling students from their classrooms, bringing them into my therapy closet, they were staring back at me, and I did not understand why they were there or what I was supposed to do with them. Just a few of the questions I was constantly asking myself were: Why are they there still? What do they need at this age? What are they not able to accomplish in the classroom that speech therapy is necessary? How does someone know they still need speech therapy? What assessment tools should be used with this age group? I had so many questions, but I did not have anyone to ask and was left trying to figure it out on my own. I had to make it work.

It is not easy being an SLP. It is even more challenging working with a new age group, one that you have little preparation for and zero guidance. This age group is different. It requires new strategies, new approaches, and a new mindset. You won't see the results of your efforts overnight. I remember working with preschoolers and seeing major growth session after session. It is harder to see that growth so quickly with this age group. There is a lot of trial-and-error. Sometimes you try one strategy and it doesn't work. So, you try something else. There were moments of frustration when a new activity or approach didn't yield immediate progress, but I learned that persistence and adaptability were key. The most rewarding part of being an SLP is seeing your students grow and succeed. When you take the time to address their root challenges, you're not just helping them survive—you're helping them thrive. You're cultivating resilience, confidence, and a stronger foundation for future growth.

WHEN I STEPPED OUT OF MY SPEECH CLOSET

I started observing my students in the classroom and the strategies used by the teachers and other providers. Most of the students on my caseload were receiving support from a reading specialist. They seemed to be targeting similar skills as I was. I observed the anchor charts that were provided to the students to help them, and I realized some things were missing. No one was addressing the core reason for their struggles. They kept practicing the skill without targeting the root cause of the problem. The anchor charts would be helpful if the students understood the vocabulary and language on them. It didn't address the *how* or the *why* the students needed these skills.

For example, I noticed an anchor chart for teaching students how to make a claim, which is a higher-level critical thinking skill. On this chart, it had an acronym to show students what to do—CLEAR—claim, evidence, and reasoning. It didn't explain what each was, how to do each step, or even show the students an example of what a successful claim would look like. If I struggled to know what to do with the chart as an SLP, I could imagine my students struggling too with it. I started having some "aha" moments.

> **TIP**
>
> This is why I created a free visual for making a claim that has question stems and is available in my TPT store at www.teacherspayteachers.com/ Product/Claim-Evidence-Reasoning-Sentence-Starters-FREEBIE- 4490356. I hung this visual on my bulletin board right by my therapy table so that my students could always see it and know exactly what was expected of them and how to verbally respond for this complicated task. It worked. They were able to use it successfully.

Moving forward, I was determined to do things differently. No guessing, no unclear expectations, no wondering how to be successful. Instead of relying on pre-made materials, I shifted to creating targeted visuals, like the claim-evidence-reasoning chart, which bridged the gap between classroom expectations and my students' actual abilities.

Over the years I have read a lot about this role and about ways to have the biggest impact. I did not like that I was unable to answer when students asked "Why am I here?" or when teachers asked "Why are you also working on that goal?"

I wanted to be able to easily and confidently explain my role and what I was doing with my students. I share with you what I have learned that has helped me explain it to others with ease.

INTRODUCING THE SCARBOROUGH READING ROPE

To be a successful reader, a student must have adequate decoding skills and language comprehension. Dr. Hollis Scarborough, a leading researcher of early language development and its connection to later literacy, developed a Reading Rope to illustrate the different components that are intertwined and interconnected in order be a skilled reader. The rope consists of two strands, lower and upper. The word-recognition strands (phonological awareness, decoding, and sight recognition of familiar words) work together for one to read fluently and become automatic. The language comprehension strands consist of background knowledge, vocabulary, language structures, verbal reasoning, and literacy knowledge. These reinforce each other and weave together with word recognition strands to produce a skilled reader. You can view a visual of this rope at www.reallygreatreading.com/blog/scarboroughs-reading-rope.

This doesn't happen overnight and requires practice. But those with language impairments require more explicit instruction to build these skills. Once you determine from language standardized assessments that there is a language impairment, you can determine how it can impact students' reading and academic success. This is why you cannot just simply create goals based on standardized subtests. You cannot have arbitrary goals. You need to make sure your goals align with how the language impairment is impacting students in the classroom or their overall communication success.

As SLPs, we also address phonological awareness skills, but for the purposes of this book, since are focusing on the upper grades, where they are reading to learn, the focus is more on the language comprehension components. Those are all our domains as speech-language pathologists. We understand language development and how these various skills are developed. We also understand that students learn in different ways and may need to be taught skills differently to grasp them and be successful. We can use graphic organizers, visual aids, sentence strips, chunking information into smaller parts, teach note-taking strategies, modeling our thinking about our thinking, visualization strategies, and more to help students learn and get those quick wins. This is our role with this age group. I go more into the specific strategies and approaches in Chapter 4. The following sections break down each of the components of the language comprehension portion of the rope more thoroughly.

Background Knowledge

Background knowledge is important to reading because it helps us make sense of new ideas and experiences. Having background knowledge gives us a significant advantage in mastering unfamiliar tasks. Studies show that when students read, they will have greater comprehension if they have background knowledge of the topic. They are better able to use context clues and, thus, achieve greater success with comprehension and vocabulary.

You can start by assessing what your students already know on a topic that you are covering. You can do this with a KWL (know, want to know, learned) chart. You can take a piece of paper and break it into three categories. Ask your student(s) what they already know about the topic and jot it down in the "know" section. Then, you can ask students what they hope to learn on the topic or what they do not know. This will go in the "W" or "want to know" column. Lastly, you can read or learn about a topic. All new information can be placed in the "learned" column.

Another way to assess is by asking students to categorize words and concepts. They can place a word or concept in the "friend" category if they are very familiar with it and can name many accurate details. They can place a word or concept in the "acquaintance" category if they are somewhat familiar with it. They may have heard of it before but cannot recall that many details. Last, they can use the "stranger" category for words and concepts they have never heard before and are unfamiliar with. By knowing how students categorize or how familiar they are, you can determine how much introduction on a topic to provide. You can use YouTube, Google Images, or even stories of your life experiences to help build their background knowledge.

Vocabulary

Vocabulary refers to the quality and quantity of words a student knows and understands. This is important for decoding and comprehending. Vocabulary can impact a student's fluency of reading. If they must continuously stop to look up words, they are likely to stop reading or not remember what they read. Students need to be able to match words they decode with words they already know the meaning of. Weak vocabulary in reading is like trying to climb a mountain with a broken compass. Without the right words to guide you, every step becomes a struggle, directions are unclear, and the path to understanding is steep and uncertain, making the journey to reading success much harder to navigate.

You can help your students build vocabulary, teach them what to do when they come across unknown words, and help them navigate texts with complex vocabulary. I discuss strategies for building vocabulary and what vocabulary words to address in the next chapter, which covers how to teach skills differently.

Language Structures

Language structures refer to syntax or the arrangement of words, or semantics, the meaning of morphemes. To read and understand, students must understand the various rules and patterns of sentences. As language structure becomes more complex and has longer sentences, students must be able to understand their meaning to get the gist of what they read. They also must understand how morphemes can change meanings.

Teaching morphemes helps students understand meanings within words. This is having an awareness of prefixes, suffixes, and base words. It is important to know what each of them mean and how they can be put together to build new words with new meanings. You have the skills and knowledge to teach students about sentence structures and how they can change meaning. You can also teach about morphemes so that they can understand new words they come across when they are familiar with their parts.

Verbal Reasoning

Verbal reasoning refers to one's ability to think about the text and infer meaning from what is explicitly and implicitly stated. This means not only understanding what was read but also reading between the lines and understanding what was not stated. Students must be able to interpret abstract language and be able to understand things like metaphors, analogies, idioms, and figurative language. If a student struggles with social inferences, this can impact their reading comprehension. They may have a difficult time understanding the perspectives of a character or they may have a difficult time following a dialogue in a text.

Literacy Knowledge

Literacy knowledge refers to understanding a text's purposes, features, and conventions. This includes understanding simple print concepts, how to hold a book, reading left to right, and letters versus sounds. Literacy knowledge also includes understanding genres of literature and that there are different types of books or texts defined by different characteristics. A skilled reader must understand the difference between fiction and nonfiction. They must be familiar with various genres like fantasy, poetry, autobiography, realistic fiction, mystery, and more. When students have a deeper understanding of literacy concepts, they will demonstrate enhanced language comprehension skills. Understanding genres helps readers anticipate the structure, themes, and typical elements of a text, leading to better comprehension and the ability to make connections within and across different types of literature. They will also improve in their ability to critically think about the texts.

By recognizing the characteristics of various genres, readers can critically evaluate the purpose, message, and style of a text, enhancing their ability to analyze and interpret meaning beyond the surface level. Navigating the world of reading without understanding literacy concepts like genres and text elements is like trying to assemble a complex puzzle without knowing what the final picture looks like. Each piece may seem random and disconnected, making it hard to see how they fit together or why they matter, leaving the reader frustrated and lost in the process.

ADDRESSING THE ROOT OF READING DIFFICULTIES

As you can see, language and reading are complicated. There are a lot of components that are necessary to be a skilled reader and demonstrate success. Language is essential in this process. There are so many necessary aspects, and most often teachers are just practicing comprehension skills and hoping for better results. No one is addressing the root of the difficulty. In many cases, the struggles of students with language impairments are treated symptomatically rather than diagnostically. Educators, specialists, and even some SLPs focus on surface-level issues—like comprehension errors, poor test performance, or disengagement—without exploring the deeper, underlying causes of these difficulties. This approach is like repeatedly patching a leaky pipe without addressing the crack itself; the immediate problem may seem resolved, but it's only a temporary fix, and the issues will continue to resurface.

Teachers and specialists often try to improve student performance by providing more practice in the same areas (e.g., repeated reading passages or comprehension questions), offering tools like anchor charts or step-by-step acronyms, or assigning more homework or drills. While well-intentioned, these strategies often fail because they don't address why the student is struggling in the first place. For example, a student who struggles with comprehension might not have the vocabulary or background knowledge to grasp the content. A student who avoids participating in class discussions may lack the syntax or verbal reasoning skills to organize their thoughts into clear sentences. A student who can't follow multistep directions might have difficulties with working memory or understanding complex sentence structures. The repeated practice of skills without identifying and resolving these foundational gaps only leads to frustration for the student and the educator.

Addressing the root of the difficulty means diving deeper into the underlying language impairments that are preventing students from succeeding. These include:

Vocabulary deficits:

- **Root issue:** Limited vocabulary impacts comprehension, fluency, and confidence in reading and speaking. Students don't understand key terms, making texts feel inaccessible.
- **Example:** A student reading a science textbook may stumble over words like "photosynthesis" or "mitochondria" because they lack prior exposure to these terms.

Weak syntax and grammar:

- **Root issue:** Students might not understand how words fit together in sentences, especially as sentence structures become more complex in secondary texts.
- **Example:** A student might struggle to parse, "Despite her protest, the experiment was continued by the researchers," because of its passive voice and subordinating conjunction.

Verbal reasoning challenges:

- **Root issue:** Difficulty making inferences, drawing conclusions, or understanding figurative language can leave students unable to answer higher-order comprehension questions.
- **Example:** A student might read a story and fail to infer a character's motivation, making it impossible to answer questions about the character's decisions.

Lack of background knowledge:

- **Root issue:** Without sufficient prior knowledge, students struggle to make connections between new information and what they already know.
- **Example:** A student reading about the Civil War might not grasp the significance of key events if they don't understand the broader historical context.

Social pragmatic deficits:

- **Root issue:** Challenges with social inference, perspective-taking, and pragmatic language affect both social interactions and reading comprehension.
- **Example:** A student may struggle to follow dialogue in a novel because they can't interpret the tone or underlying meaning of a character's words.

When these root issues aren't addressed, students may lose confidence: Repeated failures without explanation lead to avoidance behaviors or a defeatist attitude. They may fall further behind. As academic demands increase, unresolved language impairments create a widening gap between the student and their peers. They may also develop behavioral challenges. Frustration with unmet needs often manifests as disengagement, resistance, or acting out.

SLPs have the unique expertise in language and problem-solving skills to find out why students are struggling and how their language weaknesses are impacting their reading and language comprehension. Not every student can benefit from the same approach. We have this knowledge and understanding, we can impact in a different way. SLPs are uniquely equipped to address these foundational issues because of their expertise in language development and problem-solving. By identifying the root causes, SLPs can:

- **Pinpoint specific deficits:** Use assessments, observations, and informal measures to uncover where the breakdown is occurring (e.g., syntax, vocabulary, reasoning).
- **Develop targeted interventions:** Create individualized strategies that focus on building the missing skills rather than repeatedly practicing the symptoms.
- **Collaborate with other educators:** Help teachers understand the underlying challenges so they can adjust their instruction to better support the student.
- **Empower students:** Teach students strategies to overcome their language weaknesses, giving them tools to succeed independently.

Addressing the root of the difficulty isn't just about academic success—it's about changing the trajectory of a student's life. When you tackle the core challenges, you can empower students to approach learning with confidence, build meaningful connections between ideas, and advocate for themselves. When you address the root, you can get those quick wins easier and faster. As SLPs, we have the tools to make this transformation happen.

TEACHING YOUNGER VERSUS OLDER SPEECH STUDENTS

Language impairments manifest differently in older students than in younger ones, largely due to the shifting demands of school and social environments. By understanding these differences, you can better appreciate the unique challenges secondary students face and the critical role SLPs play in supporting them.

Younger students are learning to speak and to read. In early education, language development is focused on foundational skills. Younger children with language impairments often struggle with:

- **Basic communication skills:** They may have difficulty forming sentences, understanding simple instructions, or using age-appropriate vocabulary.
- **Phonological awareness:** Struggles with rhyming, segmenting, or blending sounds can hinder early reading development.
- **Building relationships:** Poor expressive and receptive skills can lead to difficulties making friends or participating in group activities.
- **Acquiring academic basics:** Challenges with early language impairments often directly impact their ability to learn letters, numbers, colors, and shapes.

The primary focus for younger students is learning the basics of communication, language, and literacy. Interventions often target early skills like articulation, sentence structure, and phonological awareness.

As students progress into secondary education, the demands placed on language skills grow significantly more complex. Language impairments in older students present differently because the expectations shift from learning to read and speak to reading, speaking, and writing to learn and express. Common challenges include the following:

Academic struggles:

- **Comprehending complex texts:** Older students are expected to read longer, more sophisticated materials that require advanced vocabulary, inference-making, and abstract thinking.
- **Critical thinking and analysis:** Tasks such as writing essays, forming arguments, and analyzing themes demand higher-level language skills that can be difficult for students with impairments.
- **Understanding academic language:** Students may struggle with discipline-specific terminology (e.g., math terms, science vocabulary) and multistep instructions.

Social and emotional challenges:

- **Navigating peer interactions:** Older students face more nuanced social expectations, such as interpreting sarcasm, reading body language, and maintaining reciprocal conversations. Language impairments can leave them feeling isolated or misunderstood.

- **Building self-esteem:** By secondary school, students are often acutely aware of their struggles and may feel "different" from their peers. This awareness can lead to frustration, avoidance, or even behavioral issues.

Transitioning to independence:

- **Preparing for life after school:** Older students need language skills to navigate interviews, write resumes, follow job instructions, and manage personal relationships. Language impairments can directly impact their ability to transition successfully into adulthood.
- **Self-advocacy:** Students with language difficulties may struggle to communicate their needs, understand their IEPs, or ask for accommodations in class or work settings.

When working with secondary students, the more you understand language's role with reading, the better advocate you can be for your students' needs. You can better explain why a student warrants speech-language therapy or does not. You can explain why you are addressing certain goals, even if another provider is doing so as well. You may both be addressing a similar need, but you will approach it from the language lens.

You can provide individualized attention and use students' strengths to overcome their weaknesses. Most teachers don't even realize this is what SLPs address. Most think we are working on articulation all day. Share the reading rope with the teachers you work with. Show them that language is essential in academic performance. SLPs are the language experts and can be an asset to the team.

You can also use this to advocate for your role with administration. Did they know that you can help improve reading and test scores? I don't want to increase your caseloads dramatically, but I do want you to get the recognition you deserve for making an impact on your students' academic successes and their lives. The more others know, the better.

GETTING PUSHBACK FROM ADMINISTRATION OR TEACHERS

I will never forget this one formal observation by my assistant principal, who was not an SLP (in my experience, they rarely are!). At the post-observation meeting, he felt the need to provide critiques, and his critique for this session was that I was reading to my students and that they should have read themselves. He felt they were passively learning. I had to explain to him that the students in the group had listening comprehension goals and that working on comprehension will help them with reading comprehension. He did not seem to grasp it and kept insisting that they weren't challenged enough. It helped me realize that I was not doing a great job of advocating for my role.

Oftentimes, when SLPs get pushback, it is due to the fact that others do not have a deep understanding of the role. They have pressures of student scores and success. They just want results and do not care how it is established. They may have had previous SLPs that just did what they were told. Whatever the reason, this section describes some ways you can respond or handle pushback. This way, if your administration questions why you are doing something, such as during a formal observation, you know how to respond.

Isn't This the Teacher's Job?

Pushback: Teachers or administrators might question why SLPs are working on comprehension, vocabulary, or other academic-like goals, assuming these are already covered in the classroom.

Why it happens: Many educators and administrators may not fully understand the scope of an SLP's role, particularly how language skills underpin academic success.

How to respond: Explain how language impairments affect a student's ability to access the curriculum, such as struggling to understand instructions, infer meaning, or use academic vocabulary effectively. Highlight that your focus is on the language foundation (e.g., syntax, verbal reasoning, morphology) that supports these classroom skills. Provide an example: "While the reading specialist works on how to decode and read fluently, I'm addressing why the student doesn't understand key vocabulary or how to formulate a complete thought in writing."

Why Are You Working on Goals the Reading Specialist Already Addresses?

Pushback: Overlap between SLP and reading specialist roles can lead to confusion or resistance.

Why it happens: There's often overlap in target areas, like comprehension or phonological awareness, but with different approaches.

How to respond: Clarify that while there may be overlap in goals, your intervention focuses on specific aspects tied to the student's language impairments. For example: "The reading specialist is working on the mechanics of reading fluency, while I'm helping the student understand figurative language or how to answer higher-order questions using reasoning skills." Offer to collaborate with the reading specialist to avoid redundancy and enhance outcomes.

Why Aren't You Working on Articulation?

Pushback: Teachers or administrators might associate SLPs primarily with articulation and question why you're addressing language-based goals instead.

Why it happens: There's often a lack of awareness about the full scope of SLP services, especially at the secondary level.

How to respond: Educate them on the range of services SLPs provide and how language impairments can directly impact academic and social success. Provide data or examples: "This student's difficulty with understanding and using complex sentence structures is making it hard for them to write essays and contribute to class discussions, which is why I'm focusing on language goals instead of articulation."

How Does This Relate to Academic Standards or Test Scores?

Pushback: Administrators may prioritize goals directly tied to standardized testing or academic benchmarks.

Why it happens: There's pressure to show measurable academic progress, and SLP goals might seem less directly tied to these metrics.

How to respond: Tie your goals to classroom success and test performance: "By addressing vocabulary and syntax, I'm helping this student improve their ability to comprehend reading passages and write cohesive responses—skills that directly impact their test scores." Share research or frameworks (like Scarborough's Reading Rope) to show how language development supports academic outcomes.

Why Are You Pulling Students Out of Class for This?

Pushback: Teachers might feel that pulling students out disrupts their learning and detracts from classroom time.

Why it happens: There's a lack of understanding about the benefits of targeted intervention or how it complements classroom instruction.

How to respond: Emphasize that your sessions are designed to address foundational skills that help students access the curriculum more effectively when they return to class. Share examples of specific improvements you've seen in similar cases, such as a student gaining confidence in classroom discussions or improving their writing skills.

Why Does This Student Still Need Speech Services?

Pushback: Administrators may question the need for continued services, especially for older students who don't present obvious speech impairments.

Why it happens: Secondary students with language goals often don't show overt signs of needing support, making it harder to justify services.

How to respond: Use clear data and observations to demonstrate the impact of language impairments on academic performance. For example: "This student's difficulty with verbal reasoning affects their ability to follow multistep directions or interpret texts, which is why continued support is necessary." Frame your services as a bridge to independence: "Our goal is to help them build skills so they no longer require this support in the future."

NOW WHAT?

Now that you have a deeper understanding of your role with older students and language's impact on reading and academic success, you can also explain this to your students when they ask, "Why am I here?" You get to explain it to them in a way they can understand. You can use the reading rope visual. Ask them what areas are difficult for them. Have those conversations so they have a better understanding of why they are there and how you can help them. The more they understand, the more buy-in they will have coming to speech, and the less they will question the value or purpose. You can then focus on addressing the weaknesses and seeing tons of progress. You can get your students a quick win by explaining the rope and its components. You can do this in the beginning of the year as part of your icebreakers and introductions, and you can always refer to it or discuss it when necessary. Have your students identify which strands are strongest and weakest for them.

As SLPs, we have a unique opportunity to create transformative change, not just in the classroom, but in the lives of the students we serve. When you focus on addressing the core language needs that underlie reading and academic success, you're doing so much more than helping students achieve their IEP goals. You're equipping them with lifelong skills that extend far beyond the walls of the school.

Every time you teach a student to decode a complex sentence, infer meaning from a text, or express their ideas with clarity and confidence, you're giving them tools they will carry into adulthood. These are the tools they'll use to advocate for themselves, to navigate relationships, to solve problems, and to participate meaningfully in society. By focusing on the foundation—language—you're building bridges that connect them to opportunities they might not have otherwise reached.

The work you do isn't easy. At times, it might feel overwhelming, especially when the progress is slow or the path forward is unclear. But it's in these moments that your expertise will shine. You are not just an interventionist; you are an advocate, problem solver, and builder of confidence. By understanding the critical connection between language and literacy, you empower your students to see what they are truly capable of achieving.

Remember, every small win—a clearer sentence, a new vocabulary word understood, a lightbulb moment in a challenging task—is a step toward something greater. With each victory, you show your students that growth is possible, that struggles can be overcome, and that their voices matter.

As you continue your journey as an SLP, embrace the role you play in your students' lives. You are not just preparing them to succeed in their next class or grade level—you are helping them navigate the world with confidence, resilience, and independence. That is the power of what SLPs do.

Now that I've broken down the essential components of language comprehension, the next step is understanding how to translate this knowledge into meaningful, individualized goals. The next chapter dives into setting realistic, impactful targets that align with your students' true needs.

CHAPTER 3

Determining Where to Start with Older Speech Students

The last chapter discussed the SLP role with older students and the impact you can have on reading. SLPs are a big deal. We can make a huge impact and help our students become confident in their learning. That is how we can get those quick wins and show our students that they can be successful. You are probably wondering where to begin. You have a student in front of you, now what? You know they have language needs based on their evaluation results. But how do you determine which goals to address? How many goals? How do you make sure you make the appropriate recommendations? The first time I sat down with my middle-school students, I was ready to tackle every language need listed in their evaluations. But as the session unfolded, it hit me: I had no idea where to start. I needed a plan—one that made sense not just on paper but for the actual students in front of me.

Why is it so difficult to determine goals for this age group? At this age, many students have been receiving speech and language services for years and/or have been struggling for years. They have numerous deficits, and it can be a challenge to know which ones to focus on.

Setting goals for middle- and high-school speech students is like trying to untangle a massive knot in a race against time. The knot represents the many challenges they face—language gaps, social communication struggles, and increasing academic demands—all tangled together after years of working on similar skills without significant breakthroughs. As they move through school, the knot tightens because academic expectations grow more complex, yet the foundational issues remain unresolved. The challenge is deciding which threads to pull first, knowing that some may take longer to untangle. You must balance addressing immediate academic needs while still working on the deeper issues, all while ensuring the student doesn't feel overwhelmed or stuck in the same place year after year.

ROLLING A GOAL OVER?

If you want to see progress, you need to set achievable goals. I remember attending a workshop early on in my career. It was run by lawyers that dealt with IEP-related cases (remember, IEPs are legal documents). They discussed the problems with "rolling over goals." I remember thinking at the time how often I saw that happen and even did it myself. The student didn't achieve the goal, so let's try again next year. Instead of rolling over, I should have considered, why didn't they achieve it? Was the goal appropriate in the first place? What did they need first to achieve that goal?

They also provided several examples such as learning the alphabet: If a student learned almost all the letters, but not all, would you roll over that goal or just anticipate they would get the rest the next year indirectly? They suggested that we wouldn't roll the goal over because we can assume they will pick up the rest of the letters incidentally, but it doesn't warrant an entire goal and an entire year to address it. They also used the example of learning to use the bathroom. That goal is so broad, and there are many skills that are needed to achieve that overarching goal of going to the bathroom. They need to know the difference between dry and wet, they need the sequence of steps, they need problem-solving skills, they need language to ask to use the bathroom, and so on. Is the goal to go to the bathroom achievable in a year if they have so many smaller objectives to accomplish? Just because we want them to achieve that goal by the end of the year, is it appropriate? You need to know the child, but most times, a broad goal like that is unachievable in a year. You need to make the goal a smaller milestone so that they can achieve it in a year.

The way I looked at goals changed tremendously after that workshop and changed the way I looked at annual goals. I needed to make sure my goals were achievable and not too broad for an entire year. That said, oftentimes SLPs inherit goals that may not be appropriate, or they make mistakes and misjudge how much a student can handle in a year.

So, what do you do if goals are not achieved by the end of the year? Instead of rolling the goal over, reconsider whether the goal is appropriate. What milestones can they achieve? How can you make the goal as specific as possible so that they can achieve it? You need to make sure you set your students up for success.

SETTING ATTAINABLE GOALS

If you pick goals randomly, your sessions will reflect it. If you don't understand what to work on, you won't see the progress you desire from your students, and they won't get those quick wins. Goals aren't just things you pluck out of thin air—though sometimes, during a hectic day, it feels like that's exactly what you're doing. You cannot just make goals based on the subtest they scored poorly on. Don't teach to the test. The more information you can gather when evaluating students or at the time you are going to write an IEP for a student, the more confident you will be to make recommendations.

Just because a student has many areas of concern doesn't mean you need to make a goal for every area. If you're setting 12 goals for one student in a year, congratulations—you've just created the Olympics of speech therapy. Let's pare it down. You only see your students once or twice a week for 30 minutes, and in groups with students working on other goals. You need to make sure the goals are attainable in the time you see them. My rule of thumb is two to three goals maximum!

Annual Versus Session Goals

Another reminder is to keep in mind that goals you set are on an annual basis. That doesn't mean you will work on that goal all year. It is what you are expecting students to achieve by the end of the IEP year. What objectives or benchmarks are necessary to meet that goal? You don't need a separate goal for every objective. But keep in mind that a goal may have some building blocks to achieve first. If you are working on the end goal all year over and over, your students will get frustrated, you will get frustrated, and you won't be successful. You need to take the time to think about where they could achievably be by the end of the year and what skills they need to be successful.

Another question to think about is, if students can't do it, what skills might they need first to then be successful with that goal? Focusing on an annual goal without teaching the benchmark skills is like trying to build a house by starting with the roof. Without a strong foundation and walls, the roof has nothing to rest on, and the entire structure is unstable. Similarly, without developing the necessary benchmark skills, the progress toward the annual goal is shaky and incomplete.

For example, if you want them to express the main idea of a passage by the end of the year, they may need to work first at the paragraph level. They may need to work on recall of significant details. They may need to recognize the vocabulary of a main idea question and know what is expected of them. They may need to know how to express the main idea in a complete sentence. All these skills may not need to be an entire IEP goal for the year but skills that can be addressed throughout the year to eventually get them to the mastery of main idea at a passage level.

Using Bloom's Taxonomy

You may have heard of Bloom's Taxonomy, which can be used to determine where your students are and what they require. Benjamin Bloom worked with other colleagues in 1956 and published a framework for categorizing educational goals. This framework was used by generations of teachers of all grade levels. Since then, this framework has developed to what is utilized today and was revised in 2001.

- The first level is "remember," which involves recalling facts and basic concepts.
- The next level is "understand," which involves explaining ideas or concepts. This includes summarizing, explaining, and interpreting.
- The next level is "apply," which involves executing and implementing.
- The next level is "analyze," which involves differentiating, organizing, and attributing.
- The next level is "evaluate," which involves critiquing, arguing, validating, predicting.
- The final level is "create," which is producing new ideas and original work from knowledge of the topic.

A classroom teacher is expected to get their students from remember to create in a unit. This may take several weeks or even months. For example, if a science teacher is working on a cell unit, they need their students to remember basic vocabulary, understand what a cell is and its parts, explain the difference between plants and animal cells, and up the hierarchy to eventually create a project with their knowledge of a cell. If a student struggles with any level of the hierarchy, they will struggle with the next level. Each level needs to be developed to progress.

As SLPs, we can use this framework for building our student's knowledge on a topic and knowing how to progress with verbal reasoning skills. Students are often expected to make inferences and predictions, so SLPs plan to work on those skills in speech therapy. However, if students can't recall what they read and don't have a deep understanding to express main ideas and summaries, they won't be able to provide verbal reasoning.

Here is using Bloom's Taxonomy with an SLP-specific examples:

- **Remember:** Identify the names of five story characters.
- **Understand:** Explain the role each character plays in the story.
- **Apply:** Predict what one character might do in a new situation.
- **Analyze:** Compare two characters' motivations.
- **Evaluate:** Argue which character made the best decision and why.
- **Create:** Write an alternate ending based on the characters' personalities.

> **TIP**
>
> I created a tool you can use to determine which level of Bloom's Taxonomy your students are at to help you create appropriate and attainable goals for them. You can access this free baseline tool with the other book resources I have for you at speechtimefun.com/book.

Picking the Right Learning Materials

That is just one piece of the puzzle to consider. You also need to be aware of your students' reading levels. You need to know what lengths and complexity they can comprehend on their own. There are several ways you can determine this:

- You can ask a reading specialist or special education teacher who may know their most recent reading levels.
- You can use reading scores on education evaluations which may indicate an age-level equivalent.

You need to determine what can they read independently, on their own without support. If you present texts that are above their reading levels, they will not comprehend what they are reading which can impact your ability to address these skills effectively.

Using materials that are too complicated for a student is like giving them a book in a foreign language they don't understand. The words may be on the page, but without the necessary background and skills, the meaning is lost, leaving them frustrated and unable to grasp the concepts. Just because a student can comprehend a specific reading level, they may have more difficulties as the text becomes longer in length. They may have difficulties recalling longer passages, impacting their ability to comprehend.

> **TIP**
>
> I created a tool that helps me determine how my students performed at different lengths and reading levels. It also helps identify what question types they can do independently, which they can do with support, and which they can't do at all. I have a critical thinking tool, which is available for free at www.speechtimefun.com/book as part of your evaluation process or to monitor students' progress.

Every Student Learns Differently

Another thing to consider when determining goals and recommendations is learning styles. Every student learns differently and has different strengths and weaknesses. You need to utilize your students' strengths to compensate for their weaknesses. You also need to teach them about their learning style and how it isn't wrong but how knowing it can help them. How can they advocate for themselves to ensure they are set up for success? You can help them understand why some approaches may be helpful to achieve complex tasks. For instance, why are you giving them a graphic organizer and maybe extra steps to write an essay?

There are many free online learning style quizzes you can do with your students. Take the quiz together and discuss the questions and what learning style means. Your students may also enjoy learning that a peer has a similar strength or weakness as they do. The more they understand, the more buy-in they will have when practicing different skills.

I like to show my students that I have weaknesses too and that they have skills that I don't have. It makes me real and relatable. They enjoy learning that I am bad at drawing or soccer since those are the things they are often strong in.

Don't Base Goals on Curriculum

Now that you understand the hierarchy and your role with reading, let's talk goals. Remember, you cannot create goals based on curriculum expectations. You need to look at the individual student and determine what are they able to achieve. Setting goals that only reflect the classroom curriculum and not the student's individual needs is like trying to fit a square peg into a round hole. No matter how much you push, it doesn't quite fit. You will end up overlooking your students' true abilities and needs. This will hinder true progress. By targeting the skills that they need and where they are, you can eventually build up to help them access the curriculum and be successful.

Instead of pulling directly from the classroom curriculum or class assignments, start by identifying the student's current language strengths and weaknesses. This is where your assessments come in. Use them to help guide you to make decisions. Your formal and informal assessments will help you uncover what underlying language skills are impacting their ability to keep up with the academic demands. Some questions to consider:

- How are the language weaknesses noted in the assessments impacting their ability to access and participate in the classroom?
- What prerequisite language concepts do they need to strengthen before they can tackle grade-level material?
- What is their current level within the language comprehension hierarchy?

By having a deeper understanding of what language concepts are necessary and where they are currently performing, you can make confident, individualized recommendations for goals that will ultimately support access to the curriculum. This approach will lead to more meaningful progress and empower students with the tools they need to succeed both in the classroom and beyond.

SMART Goals Reminder

Just a friendly reminder of SMART goals, which is a framework used to create clear, concise, and achievable objectives. The acronym SMART stands for specific, measurable, achievable, relevant, and time-bound.

Goals should be clear and specific, addressing the "who, what, where, when, and why" of the objective. This ensures that the goal is well-defined and unambiguous. Goals need to be measurable so that progress can be tracked. This involves setting criteria for what success looks like and how it will be quantified (e.g., percentage, frequency, accuracy). Goals should be realistic and attainable, considering the student's current abilities and resources. Setting achievable goals ensures that the student is challenged but not overwhelmed. Goals should be relevant to the student's needs and aligned with broader educational objectives. Goals should have a clear timeframe, specifying when the objective should be met. This creates a sense of urgency and helps prioritize the steps needed to achieve the goal. Think about a student you're working with right now. Are their goals specific enough? Achievable in the time you see them? What foundational skills might they need first?

Some friendly tips to ensure that your goals are SMART:

- First, before writing the goal, assess the student's current abilities to establish a baseline. This will help you create a goal that is challenging yet attainable.
- Second, ensure that the goals are relevant to the student's everyday communication needs. This makes the goals more meaningful and applicable to real-life situations.
- Third, break down large goals. If a goal seems too broad, break it down into smaller, more manageable benchmarks. This allows for more targeted instruction and clearer progress tracking.
- Last, use positive language. Focus on what the student will achieve rather than what they need to avoid or stop doing. This promotes a growth mindset and encourages motivation.

The better the goal, the easier it is to understand, easier it is to know where to start, and easier it is to collect data and notice progress. If the goal is unclear, your path will be unclear as well. Take one of your current student's goals and break it down: What smaller steps do they need to achieve first? Are you addressing those building blocks?

When You Receive an IEP from Another SLP

A challenge secondary SLPs often face is receiving students with IEPs written previously by another SLP. Maybe they came from another school or transferred from another district. Sometimes we have access to reports, sometimes we only have access to the IEPs. Every state and district have different protocols for new entrants, but most of the time districts must hold a meeting to make sure the IEP is developed for the district they are in. Regardless, if the IEP came from your district, your colleague across the hall, or someone across the country, you may not understand their recommendations or agree with them. Sometimes, inherited IEP goals feel like a scavenger hunt where the clues don't quite add up. What was this SLP thinking? Did they have a secret code you missed?

I always like to probe and find out for myself if the goals are appropriate and attainable for that student. Are there too many goals? What are they stimulable for? Is a goal reflective of where they are or what they can achieve? Just like you would use the various tools and frameworks to determine goals and where to start if these were your students from the get-go, you can use them to determine if the goals you inherited are appropriate. You can amend goals that aren't appropriate. You can ask an administrator or case manager what the protocol is for your state or district.

Just because a goal was written, doesn't mean you have to agree with it. You want to make sure you set your students up for success. This is why you also need to be mindful when writing IEPs that you might not be the one working with the student in the future. Don't include certain programs or tools that may not be clear or accessible to the next therapist.

Common Goal Mistakes

We have all made these mistakes. But let's put them out there and promise to do better.

Setting Too Many Goals

It's tempting to write goals for every area of weakness identified in evaluations, but too many goals can overwhelm both the student and the SLP.

Example: Writing six goals for a student who struggles with vocabulary, grammar, social skills, auditory comprehension, articulation, and fluency.

Why it's a problem:

- Splits focus, leading to limited progress in any one area
- Makes it difficult to provide meaningful intervention during limited session times
- Increases the workload for progress monitoring and documentation

The fix:

- Prioritize: Select two or three high-impact goals that will address core weaknesses and support other skills.
- Think globally: Choose goals that have a ripple effect (e.g., improving vocabulary can also help with reading comprehension and verbal expression).

Focus on fewer, stronger goals—it's better to make meaningful progress in two areas than superficial progress in six.

Setting Goals That Are Too Broad or Vague

I highly recommend that you avoid writing goals that are too general or don't specify measurable outcomes.

Example: "The student will improve reading comprehension skills."

Why it's a problem:

- Lacks clarity on what progress looks like
- Makes it difficult to track improvement or justify success
- Leaves room for interpretation, which can lead to inconsistency in implementation

The fix:

- Use SMART criteria (specific, measurable, achievable, relevant, time-bound).
- Break down broad goals into specific, observable objectives.
- Example of a SMART goal: "By the end of the school year, the student will identify the main idea of a fictional paragraph with 80% accuracy in four out of five trials."

Vague goals are like vague directions—no one knows where they're going or how to get there.

Ignoring Foundational Skills

We may be tempted to just go straight to working on higher-level skills. However, we must remember to first address underlying weaknesses.

Example: Working on predicting outcomes when the student can't yet recall key details from a passage.

Why it's a problem:

- Leads to frustration for the student, who struggles without the necessary building blocks
- Results in slow or no progress because the foundation isn't solid

The fix:

- Identify prerequisite skills and address those first.
- Use frameworks like Bloom's Taxonomy to scaffold learning.
- Example: If the goal is to summarize a passage, start with identifying key details in sentences, then paragraphs, before moving to full passages.

Skipping foundational skills is like trying to bake a cake without mixing the ingredients—it just doesn't hold together.

Focusing Only on Test Scores

When determining goals, rather than basing them solely on standardized test results, consider functional needs or classroom impact.

Example: Writing a goal to improve synonyms because of a low test score, even though the student struggles more with answering questions in class discussions.

Why it's a problem:

- Test scores don't always reflect the skills students need to succeed in real-life settings.
- Goals may not address areas most relevant to the student's academic and social performance.

The fix:

- Look beyond test scores—consider teacher input, parent concerns, classroom performance, and observations.
- Write goals that bridge the gap between testing and functional needs (e.g., vocabulary building for better class participation).

A goal based only on test scores is like fixing a flat tire when the engine is what's stalling the car.

Writing Overcomplicated Goals

Avoid writing goals that are overly complex or involve multiple skills at once.

Example: "The student will independently use context clues to determine the meaning of unknown words in grade-level texts while summarizing the main idea with 90% accuracy."

Why it's a problem:

- Combines multiple objectives, making it harder to track progress
- Overwhelms students and can lead to slower progress

The fix:

- Break down complex goals into smaller, focused steps.
- Example: "The student will identify context clues to determine the meaning of unknown words with 80% accuracy" (Addressing summarizing as a separate goal).

Keep goals focused—trying to do too much at once is like juggling chainsaws; it's bound to go sideways.

Setting Unrealistic Goals

Avoid writing goals that are too ambitious for the student's current skill level or the time available.

Example: Expecting a student with severe expressive language delays to compose a five-paragraph essay within one year.

Why it's a problem:

- Sets the student up for failure, which can harm their confidence
- Causes frustration for both the SLP and the student

The fix:

- Consider the student's baseline performance and set incremental, achievable goals. Example: Start with single-sentence formulation before advancing to paragraphs.
- Use SMART criteria to ensure the goal is both realistic and challenging.

A goal should stretch students, but not so far that they snap.

Basing Goals on Curriculum Alone

Avoid setting goals based on grade-level standards instead of the student's individual abilities.

Example: Writing a goal to master grade-level text analysis for a student who reads significantly below grade level.

Why it's a problem:

- Overlooks the student's actual needs and creates unrealistic expectations
- Prioritizes compliance over meaningful progress

The fix:

- Focus on the student's current skill level and functional needs.
- Create goals that help the student build toward accessing the curriculum over time, rather than meeting it immediately.
- Example: "The student will recall key details from a grade-appropriate paragraph with 80% accuracy in three out of four trials."

The curriculum is the destination, but goals are the steps to get there—meet the student where they are.

Failing to Collaborate

Avoid writing goals without input from teachers, parents, or the student themselves.

Why it's a problem:

- Misses critical insights about the student's needs and strengths
- Risks writing goals that don't align with classroom expectations or real-world challenges

The fix:

- Collaborate during IEP meetings and evaluations.
- Ask teachers what skills would benefit the student most in class.
- Involve the student by asking what they want to improve or where they feel they struggle.

Collaboration turns a good goal into a great one—because everyone is rowing in the same direction.

Using Negative Language

Avoid using negative language and avoid focusing on what the student can't do or needs to stop doing.

Example: "The student will stop making grammatical errors when speaking."

Why it's a problem:

- Can be demotivating for students and parents
- Shifts the focus away from growth and toward deficits

The fix:

- Use positive, growth-oriented language.
- Example: "The student will use correct subject-verb agreement in four out of five opportunities during structured conversations."

Goals should be a roadmap to success, not a list of what's wrong.

Not Revisiting Goals Regularly

It can be easy to set goals and forget them. Avoid setting goals at the beginning of the year and never revisiting them until progress reports are due.

Why it's a problem:

- Misses opportunities to adjust goals based on progress or changes in needs
- Can lead to irrelevant or stagnant goals if circumstances change

The fix:

- Schedule regular check-ins to assess progress.
- Be flexible—modify goals if they're no longer appropriate or achievable.

Goals aren't set in stone—they're a living plan that grows with the student.

By addressing these common mistakes, you can ensure your students' goals are effective, and actionable, and you set your students up for success.

FIXING BAD GOALS

This section includes examples of how you can adjust wording to make your goals better.

Bad goal: "The student will improve reading comprehension."

Why it's bad:

- Vague and lacks specificity
- No measurable criteria or timeframe

Good goal: "By the end of the academic year, the student will identify the main idea of a fictional paragraph with 80% accuracy in three out of four trials, as measured by SLP observation."

Why it's good:

- Specifies the task (main idea), accuracy level (80%), and context (fictional paragraphs)
- Includes a measurable timeframe and how progress will be assessed

Bad goal: "The student will improve sentence structure."

Why it's bad:

- Too broad and non-specific
- Does not describe what "improvement" looks like

Good goal: "By the end of the IEP year, the student will verbally produce compound sentences using conjunctions (e.g., and, but, because) in four out of five opportunities during structured therapy tasks, as measured by SLP observation."

Why it's good:

- Focuses on a specific skill (compound sentences with conjunctions)
- States the accuracy level and measurement method

Bad goal: "The student will improve their /r/ sound."

Why it's bad:

- No details about context, accuracy, or timeframe
- Vague about what "improve" means

Good goal: "By the end of the IEP period, the student will produce the /r/ sound in all word positions with 90% accuracy across three consecutive therapy sessions, as measured by SLP data collection."

Why it's good:

- Specifies the sound (/r/), context (word positions), and accuracy level (90%)
- Includes a clear measurement and timeframe

Bad goal: "The student will learn new words."

Why it's bad:

- Lacks specificity about how many words, what type of words, or how progress will be tracked

Good goal: "By the end of the academic year, the student will use context clues to determine the meaning of 10 Tier 2 vocabulary words with 80% accuracy in four out of five trials, as measured by SLP observation."

Why it's good:

- Clearly defines the skill (using context clues), the word type (Tier 2), and the accuracy level
- Provides a measurable outcome and timeframe

Bad goal: "The student will answer questions after listening to a story."

Why it's bad:

- Vague about what type of questions, how many, or the context
- No measurable criteria

Good goal: "By the end of the school year, the student will answer literal WH questions (e.g., who, what, where) after listening to a three- or four-sentence story with 80% accuracy in four out of five trials, as measured by SLP data collection."

Why it's good:
Specifies the type of question (literal WH), context (three- or four-sentence story), and accuracy level
Includes a timeframe and assessment method

Bad goal: "The student will speak more fluently."

Why it's bad:

- Too broad and subjective
- Lacks measurable criteria or specifics about the skill being targeted

Good goal: "By the end of the IEP year, the student will use a learned fluency strategy (e.g., slow rate, easy onset) to decrease stuttering episodes during a two-minute conversation to no more than three disfluencies, as measured by SLP data."

Why it's good:

- Specifies the skill (fluency strategy) and desired outcome (no more than three disfluencies)
- Includes context (two-minute conversation) and method of measurement

Bad goal: "The student will improve perspective-taking skills."

Why it's bad:

- Vague and doesn't define what "improve" means or how it will be assessed
- Lacks specificity about the skill or context

Good goal: "By the end of the school year, the student will identify how another person might feel in a given social scenario (e.g., being excluded from a group activity) and explain why in four out of five opportunities, as measured by SLP observation."

Why it's good:

- Clearly defines the skill (identifying feelings and providing an explanation)
- Specifies the context (social scenarios) and measurable criteria (four out of five opportunities)
- Aligns with real-world social interactions

Hopefully after reading these examples, you can see how you can adjust your goals or use these as a starting point when coming up with your own goals. These examples highlight the importance of specificity, measurability, and relevance in creating effective goals that support meaningful progress. The stronger the goal, the easier it is to have quick wins!

INTERPRETING TEST RESULTS AND SETTING APPROPRIATE GOALS

Now that you have a deeper understanding of why relevant and appropriate goals are important, this section shares some examples of how to interpret results and determine goals from them.

Student name: Alex
Grade: 7 (middle school)
Test administered: Clinical Evaluation of Language Fundamentals, 5th Edition (CELF-5)

Subtest scores:
Receptive Language Index: 75 (low average)
Expressive Language Index: 68 (below average)
Core Language Score: 70 (below average)

Understanding Spoken Paragraphs: 6th percentile
Word Definitions: 4th percentile
Formulated Sentences: 5th percentile

Summary: Alex's CELF-5 results indicate significant difficulty with expressive language, particularly in formulating sentences and defining words. Alex also struggles with understanding spoken paragraphs, which affects his ability to comprehend and respond to classroom instructions effectively.

Goals based on the results: By the end of the academic year, Alex will accurately formulate complete sentences using appropriate subject-verb agreement four out of five times in structured therapy sessions, as measured by SLP observation.

By the end of the academic year, Alex will accurately use context clues to determine meanings of unknown Tier 2 vocabulary words three out of five times in structured therapy sessions, as measured by SLP observation.

Let's break this down: The goals target sentence formulation and vocabulary, which are areas of weakness identified in the CELF-5. The goals are directly relevant to the challenges Alex faces, particularly in expressive language, which impacts his academic success. These goals ensures that Alex receives targeted intervention in areas that are directly impacting his ability to succeed in the classroom.

Student name: Maria
Grade: 10 (high school)
Test administered: Comprehensive Assessment of Spoken Language, 2nd Edition (CASL-2)

Subtest scores:
Synonyms: 85 (low average)
Sentence Expression: 78 (below average)
Grammaticality Judgment: 75 (below average)
Idiomatic Language: 70 (below average)
Pragmatic Judgment: 82 (low average)

Summary: Maria's CASL-2 results indicate significant difficulty with understanding and using idiomatic language, as well as challenges with sentence expression and grammatical accuracy. These deficits affect her ability to comprehend and produce language that is often required in high school-level academic tasks, such as essay writing, understanding literature, and engaging in complex classroom discussions.

Relevant speech therapy goal based on CASL-2 results: By the end of the school year, Maria will improve her ability to understand and use idiomatic expressions using context clues 7 out of 10 trials, as measured by SLP observation.

By the end of the school year, Maria will verbally express compound sentences using conjunctions three out of five trials in structured therapy sessions, as measured by SLP observation.

Let's break this one down: The goals target idiomatic language and sentence structure, which are areas of weakness identified in the CASL-2. The goals are directly relevant to Maria's challenges, particularly in areas critical for high school success, such as understanding complex texts and expressing ideas clearly. These goals are designed to help Maria develop the language skills necessary for her academic success in high school.

These are just two examples of how you can take test results, evaluate how the skills assessed will impact performance in the classroom, and create goals based on them. Notice, I did not create a goal for every weakness. Keep it simple. Keep it achievable. Keep it relevant. This is how we make our sessions relevant without having to use the curriculum. We are helping students access the curriculum.

I once had a student that struggled to summarize even short paragraphs. Instead of starting with "summarize the main idea of a passage," we began by identifying key details in single sentences. Once she mastered that, we moved to two-sentence paragraphs. By the end of the year, this student could confidently summarize a full passage—and even started helping her classmates! We didn't work on her end goal the entire year, we worked up to it. We got quick wins and built confidence at the same time.

Remember the Subtests Are a Snapshot

Remember that standardized tests are just a snapshot of how a student is performing. The manuals provide detailed explanations of what each subtest is assessing and what the results indicate. I get it—we have to use standardized tests for billing and qualifying purposes. It also does give us some valuable information. But it is just a starting point. Tests offer a structured, consistent way to measure language skills, but they don't tell us the entire story. These tests are typically administered quickly in controlled environments with limited distractions, and they often focus on isolated tasks that don't always reflect dynamic, real-world demands of the classroom.

A student might score within normal limits on a standardized test, but still struggle to keep up with classroom discussions, understand grade-level texts, or express their thoughts clearly in writing. On the flip side, a student may perform poorly on a test due to anxiety, attention challenges, or unfamiliar test formats, even if they have strong functional skills in daily academic settings. This is why we cannot stop at the test scores. To truly understand a student's language capabilities, we need to look beyond what that one single test provides. What does this mean? We need to observe them in different settings. We need to gather input from teachers, parents, and the students themselves. We need to utilize informal assessments, language samples, and dynamic assessments to see how the student performs with support or real tasks. We need to always be considering executive functioning, motivation, attention, and the student's interests and learning styles.

When we combine the snapshot from the standardized testing with this richer, more holistic picture, we can develop goals and plans that are not only accurate, but actually meaningful and motivating to the student.

NOW WHAT?

If you walk away with one major understanding from this chapter, I hope it is to make sure the goal is appropriate for the student in front of you, not what they are expected to achieve for their age or grade. The better the goal and the more achievable it is, the easier it will be to teach it, collect data, see progress, and eventually document and write progress reports.

SLPs often have large caseloads with overflowing paperwork. The clearer the goals, the easier the rest will be. Take a moment to reflect on the goals your students have and the materials you are currently using with them. Do you understand the rationale for them and why they were generated in the first place? Could any goals be amended? Do you know your students' reading levels? Are you using materials at their reading levels? Maybe you can make a quick plan to find out the reading levels or ask the previous SLP why they generated those goals.

The more you understand, the easier it will be to determine how to teach your students so they can get those quick wins. Now it's your turn. Reflect on one of your students. Are their goals clear, attainable, and impactful? If not, what changes will you make today to set them up for success? Remember, the better the goals, the bigger the wins—for them and for you.

The next chapter explains how to teach these skills so that you can get those quick wins and build your students' confidence.

CHAPTER 4

Teaching Strategies and Techniques

The previous chapters discussed your role in reading and academic success and the huge impact language comprehension has. They discussed different tools to use to know how to determine where to start. But now, you have these students in front of you, and they have these language comprehension goals.

When I started with older students, I just grabbed any worksheet or game that worked on that goal. I found workbooks for the grade level, and I would just print or photocopy and go. There weren't any speech-specific activities, but I found worksheets for English language arts or reading comprehension. I would keep practicing these skills based on the goals given to me. Sometimes students would seem to get it. Sometimes they wouldn't. I would then just find more practice games and worksheets. I kept presenting these activities. I tried to make it fun. I tried to turn it into a game.

Although I was getting the job done, I didn't feel effective. I didn't see progress. I didn't see excitement, and I wasn't excited either. Then I had an "aha" moment. If I was using reading and ELA worksheets and books, weren't those professionals also using these? Why would students need to do this with me? How was I different? Why wasn't this practice enough with those teachers? I started thinking about what I was doing when completing these tasks. What was I innately doing? What kind of questions was I asking myself to achieve these tasks? What skills did I need to be successful? What did I need to know to answer these comprehension questions?

One of my favorite quotes is from Albert Einstein, "Insanity is doing the same things over and over again and expecting different results." We often find ourselves stuck in this. We often work on the annual goal all year long and wonder why our students are frustrated and not making progress. Chapter 3 mentioned that we need to consider different milestones and benchmarks that will help our students get to that annual goal. We also need to consider that they may have already been taught these skills or been exposed to these concepts in the classroom, but they didn't stick. Students are still unable to grasp them. We need a different approach. Let's face it—if your strategy feels like it came from the depths of a dusty ELA workbook, your students have already checked out. We've all been there.

Determining your students' learning styles is a great place to start. You can use their strengths to tap into their weaknesses. If they are visual learners, consider how you can enhance the visual supports to compensate for their auditory weaknesses. If they are auditory learners, consider how you can reduce the visual stimuli and enhance their ability to listen for key words, recognize when they get distracted and need information again, and what to do if there is excessive background noise. The more you teach your students about their strengths and how the strategies you are teaching them will help them, the more they will understand the value of being in your speech room. They will understand the benefit and want to participate. Don't be afraid to discuss it regularly. They benefit from repetition.

This chapter discusses several strategies to target and teach differently. You also need to explicitly teach the different strategies. If you could simply give a student a strategy and expect them to be successful, they would have been successful in the classroom. Someone has determined that they can benefit from individualized, explicit instruction. This is how you provide it.

USING GRAPHIC ORGANIZERS

Let's start with my favorite strategy of using graphic organizers. There are so many benefits of using graphic organizers to improve language comprehension. Graphic organizers help students break down and visualize complex language structures, making it easier to comprehend and retain information from challenging texts or spoken language. Graphic organizers reduce cognitive overload by breaking down complex information into manageable parts. This visual aid allows students to focus on one piece of information at a time, making it easier to process and retain without feeling overwhelmed by the overall complexity of the material. By organizing information visually, students can better identify relationships between ideas, which promotes deeper critical thinking and analysis of the material being studied or discussed. Think of graphic organizers as the ultimate cheat sheet—there's no shame in making life easier for you and your students.

Using graphic organizers can help students clarify their thoughts before speaking, leading to more confident and coherent verbal communication during discussions, presentations, or everyday conversations. Graphic organizers help students structure their thoughts and ideas before writing, leading to clearer, more logically organized written responses. Written language is language, and you can support them here as well. This tool allows them to map out their main points, supporting details, and conclusions, resulting in well-structured and cohesive essays or answers. Let's consider some examples of graphic organizers.

Examples

If you are working at the basic recall level, you can utilize a graphic organizer to help students focus their reading or listening. They can listen for the key story elements: character, setting, problem, solution.

If you are working on identifying and expressing main ideas and being able to get the gist of a text, you can have students identify significant details and then use them to determine the main idea.

For summarizing, this depends on if the narrative is fiction or nonfiction. All narrative texts can be summarized using the terms: Somebody, Wanted, But, So, Then. This will help students focus on the key elements and what is important to recall and express. It also helps them focus only on relevant information and filter out unnecessary details. This helps them provide a more elaborate response than just the sequence of events.

For example, if summarizing *Shrek*, one can respond with "The movie Shrek was about an ogre name Shrek that wanted a peaceful swamp. But, fairy tale creatures came and took over his swamp. So, he went to visit Lord Farquaad and asked for his swamp back. Then, Lord Farquaad sent him to save Princess Fiona, and they fell in love and lived happily ever after."

I love using familiar movies and stories to model how to use this strategy. For nonfiction texts, I like to have students listen for and identify the main idea, the author's purpose for writing the text, and two to three significant details related to the main idea that they learned. For making predictions or making inferences, I like to have students look or listen for clues in the text or evidence they can prove, refer to their background knowledge, and make guesses or predictions based on their evidence and background knowledge. These are just some of the several examples of graphic organizers I like to use to teach students what to focus on while reading or listening and know what is expected of them to respond.

Teaching with Graphic Organizers

How do you teach students with graphic organizers? First, determine the goal or focus of the lesson. Then, determine the graphic organizer that will best meet their needs. Do they need more visuals? Less complexity? Prompts or examples on how to complete it? I like to use the "I do" "we do" "you do" approach with graphic organizers.

Remember, if you can just give a graphic organizer to a student and expect them to be successful, you could have just provided it to the teacher. Plus, they may have already been exposed to these. You need to model or "I do." Explicitly show your thinking about your thinking. How do you question yourself and stop and think about when to jot down responses? Do you need to stop after a page, a paragraph, or even a sentence? What questions do you ask yourself?

Then, you can do it together, or "we do." Maybe you provide scaffolds like the answers that will go inside the Venn diagram, and students must determine where they go. Maybe you use cloze sentences or fill-in-the blank sentences for them to complete with you as they utilize the graphic organizer. Last, they can try it on their own. Remember, this won't be all in one session. This can take several sessions, and that's okay since it's an annual goal after all.

Once we have students using graphic organizers to support them, we must show them how they can use this skill in the classroom. How will this help them? Make sure you share the specific graphic organizers with their teachers and support staff working with them, so that everyone is aware and utilizing the same tools to support them. You don't want their teachers utilizing a different version of a graphic organizer because that can impact their carry-over and success.

TEACHING NOTE-TAKING STRATEGIES

Students are often expected to take notes. The problem is that they don't know what to write, don't know how to refer to notes, and then won't use notes because they don't find them helpful. You need to explicitly teach them how to take notes and how to refer to them. If students are successful at the paragraph level but struggle to recall and comprehend when the texts become longer and more complex, a note-taking or chunking strategy can be beneficial. If you're reading instructions for assembling furniture or following a recipe, breaking it into steps helps you stay organized and avoid mistakes.

You can teach students to stop after each paragraph, or sentence if that is where they are at, and prompt themselves with questions to check for understanding and recall. Did they understand what they just read? I like to teach students to think about the main idea. This shows they get the gist and gives them a simple sentence or phrase to jot down in the margins. You can also teach them to use sticky notes if the margins are too small or too busy for them. For a fictional text, they can ask "Who or what was it about and what happened to them?" For a nonfiction text, "What was it about and what did you learn?"

Once they can master the main idea of the paragraphs and are able to jot them down, you need to teach them how to refer to the text. These students struggle with reading and may not know how to skim a text to locate their answers. You need to teach them to read or listen to a question, determine a key word that is being asked of them, and look at their jotted notes to find which paragraph is about what the question is referring to. Then, you can teach them to reread the paragraph to determine their responses. This makes it less overwhelming then to reread the entire text again to locate their evidence or determine how to respond.

Color-Coding Note-Taking Strategy

You can introduce color-coding with note-taking. Color-coding involves assigning specific colors to different types of information in a text, notes, or graphic organizers. The goal is to create a visual hierarchy that helps students quickly identify and organize critical details, making it easier to recall and review later.

Color-coding is effective because it leads to:

- **Visual organization:** Students can quickly differentiate between types of information, such as main ideas, details, and vocabulary.
- **Memory support:** Visual learners retain color-coded information more easily than plain text.
- **Reduced cognitive load:** Separating information by color helps students focus on one category at a time.
- **Improved recall:** Associating colors with specific types of information creates a mental shortcut for retrieving details.

Follow these steps to teach the color-coding technique:

Step 1: Assign Colors to Categories

- Choose colors that are visually distinct and easy to remember.
- Examples of categories:
    - **Main ideas:** Use a bold color like blue or green.
    - **Key details or supporting evidence:** Use yellow or orange.
    - **Unfamiliar vocabulary:** Use pink or purple.
    - **Questions or unclear information:** Use red for items that require follow-up.

Step 2: Model the Process

- Provide an example text and demonstrate how to highlight or underline information using the assigned colors.
- Think aloud as you highlight:
  - "This sentence is the main idea of the paragraph, so I'll mark it in blue."
  - "This word is new to me, so I'll underline it in pink to remind myself to look it up later."

Step 3: Guided Practice

- Have students work on a short passage with you, color-coding together as you guide them through identifying categories.

Step 4: Independent Practice

- Gradually release responsibility, allowing students to practice color-coding independently on increasingly complex texts.

Uses of Color-Coding

- **Note-taking in texts, using highlighting or underlining:** Provide students with a passage and assign them a task, such as identifying the main idea, key details, and unfamiliar words using the assigned colors.
- **Graphic organizers:** Use colored pens or markers to fill in sections of a graphic organizer. Example: In a "Somebody, Wanted, But, So, Then" graphic organizer, use different colors for each section to make it visually distinct.
- **Summarizing:** Assign colors to parts of a summary. Main ideas are in one color, supporting details in another, and any unanswered questions in a third color.
- **Vocabulary building:** Use color-coded flashcards. Write the vocabulary word in one color and the definition in another. Use a third color for an example sentence.
- **Tracking progress:** During sessions, students can use color-coded sticky notes to mark tasks they've mastered, need help with, or find challenging.

Tools for Color-Coding

Digital tools:

- **Google Docs or Slides:** Use the highlighter tool or text colors to implement color-coding digitally.
- **Notion or Evernote:** Create color-coded tags or highlights in digital notes.

Physical tools:

- **Colored pens or highlighters:** Assign specific pens or markers to different categories.
- **Sticky notes:** Use sticky notes in different colors to annotate physical texts.

Tips for Success

- **Keep it simple:** Start with two or three categories and add more as students become comfortable.
- **Make it consistent:** Use the same colors for the same categories across texts to build familiarity.
- **Teach self-monitoring:** Encourage students to pause periodically and check if their notes are clear and well-organized.
- **Customize for students:** Adapt the categories and colors based on individual student needs.

Benefits of Color-Coding for Students

- Encourages active engagement with texts and materials
- Builds organizational skills that transfer to academic tasks like essay writing or test preparation
- Reduces anxiety when reviewing complex information, as the colors simplify what to focus on

TEACHING THE CHUNKING STRATEGY

Chunking is a great strategy for students who get overwhelmed when they see a longer text. Another way to use chunking is to only present one paragraph at a time to reduce overwhelm. You can do this several ways:

- You can take scissors and cut the text into pieces so that each piece has a paragraph. You can present each paragraph at a time.
- Another way is to recreate the text. Either type it into a new document or copy and paste it if it is a digital text. Enlarge the text so that each page only has one paragraph. You can present the student with one page or paragraph at a time and check for understanding before providing the new paragraph or page.
- You can also chunk digitally by putting each paragraph on a Google Slide page.
- You can even use a table to provide a note-taking spot for students to jot down their main ideas.

You can try all these methods with your students and see which they prefer and respond best to.

TEACHING METACOGNITIVE THINKING

Metacognitive thinking is thinking about thinking. This requires students to think internally, self-question, and self-reflect. This requires internal dialogue, which is language. You can explicitly teach your students how to do this and its benefits. There are many benefits to teaching this:

- Metacognition helps students become aware of their own thought processes, enabling them to recognize when they understand the material and when they need to employ strategies to improve comprehension.
- By thinking about their thinking, students can better identify gaps in their understanding. They can be more aware of what they don't know and apply specific strategies to overcome challenges, leading to better problem-solving skills.
- Metacognitive strategies often involve techniques for organizing and summarizing information, which can improve students' ability to retain and recall information over time.
- Over time, the consistent use of metacognitive strategies can lead to improved performance in academic tasks that require strong language comprehension skills.

So how do you do this? You can model your thinking about your thinking. You can show students how you do this without even realizing it and how it can support them. Provide them with scripts that they can use for themselves. Practice it out loud in various situations. Encourage students to ask themselves questions as they read or listen to information. Questions like "What is the main idea?" "Do I understand this part?" and "What should I do if I don't?" guide students to actively monitor their comprehension and adjust their strategies as needed.

The following sections go through several examples for how to do this with your students.

Think-Aloud While Reading a Complex Text

Example: "As I'm reading this paragraph, I notice that I'm starting to get confused about what the author is trying to say. Let me go back and reread the last sentence to see if that helps. Hmm, it still doesn't make sense. Maybe I need to look at the context or see if there's a key word that might clarify the meaning. I'll also underline the parts that are confusing so I can ask about them later."

Problem-Solving During a Difficult Task

Example: "I'm working on this math problem, but I'm not sure what to do next. Let me pause and think about what I already know. The problem is asking for the total, so I need to add these two numbers. But before I do that, I'll double-check the steps to make sure I'm not missing anything important. If I'm still stuck, I can look back at a similar problem we solved earlier or ask for help."

Planning and Monitoring a Writing Assignment

Example: "I have to write an essay, and I'm thinking about how to start. First, I'll brainstorm some ideas and jot them down. Now, I'll organize these ideas into an outline. As I write, I'll keep checking my outline to make sure I'm staying on track. If I notice that I'm getting off-topic or my ideas aren't flowing well, I'll stop and see what needs to be adjusted. After I finish, I'll review the essay to ensure that I met all the requirements and that it's clear and well-organized."

By providing your students models of your own thought process, they can see the benefits and be able to use the models to incorporate these strategies for themselves. You need to explicitly teach them how and what they can get from it as a result. You want them to see those quick wins and that they can be successful.

You can also provide more role-playing activities. Have students practice being "thinking coaches" for one another, guiding their peers through self-questioning strategies.

USING VISUAL AIDS

Many students we work with are visual learners. They can benefit from visual supports to enhance their understanding of written and oral language. You can use pictures, videos, diagrams, or physical objects to support understanding of abstract or unfamiliar concepts and help make these concepts more concrete and relatable. Teachers often use anchor charts as visuals to teach new vocabulary or concepts. You can use the same concept but be more specific about what is expected of them and show them steps to achieve a task or even visual representations of new vocabulary. You don't need fancy anchor charts or large posters. You can be effective with paper-sized visuals or even index cards. Use apps like Canva or Google Slides to build custom visuals tailored to individual student goals.

There are many benefits to using visuals to help students comprehend new concepts:

- Visual aids make abstract concepts more concrete, helping students better grasp and retain information.
- Incorporating visual elements can help capture a student's attention. This can improve their engagement by making sessions more interactive and less monotonous.
- Visuals can help improve memory and recall since visuals are processed more easily and stored longer in memory.
- For students with language difficulties, visual aids provide an alternative way to express ideas. This can reduce frustration and improve communication.
- By breaking down information into visual components, students can focus on one aspect at a time, reducing the cognitive effort required to understand complex material. Repeated exposure to visual aids reinforces key concepts and skills. This helps students internalize and apply what they've learned.
- Lastly, visual aids support multisensory learning. They complement auditory information, engaging multiple senses and supporting students with different learning preferences.

Here are some examples of visual supports that you can use with your students to support their needs and improve their comprehension and understanding:

Story sequencing cue cards: You can use picture cards to help students understand the sequence of events in a story. You can have a different card that represents a different part of the narrative. This will allow students to visually organize the story from beginning to end. This can also help with retrieval of information and help them express the sequence of events in order with less cognitive overload.

Vocabulary flashcards with images: You can introduce new vocabulary words using flashcards that pair the word with a relevant image. This helps students connect the word with its meaning, improving retention and understanding. I recommend using real photos from Google Images or such sources. You don't want the pictures to be so "cutesy" that your students won't want to use them. Although I previously discussed the graphic organizer for summarizing narrative texts, you can also provide a visual support to remind them of the strategy to listen for and express using the terms: Somebody, Wanted, But, So, Then.

PROVIDING SENTENCE STARTERS OR CARRIER PHRASES

SLPs can use sentence starters or carrier phrases to support students in recalling information and improving language comprehension by providing a structured way to organize their thoughts and responses.

> **NOTE**
>
> Sentence starters and carrier phrases are structure prompts that help students initiate or organize their thoughts when speaking or writing. A sentence starter is the beginning of a sentence that guides students in how to respond (i.e., "I think that. . ." "The main idea is. . ." "One example is. . ."). Carrier phrases are repeated frames that stay the same while students fill in the key information (i.e. "I see a ____." "This is a ___ because ____."). Both tools can reduce the cognitive load for your students, provide a scaffold for expressive language, and help students participate more confidently in academic tasks while building sentence structure and vocabulary skills.

You can support your students with sentence starters or carrier phases using sentence strips, sticky notes, index cards, visually on a worksheet, or even written on a dry erase board. You can go even crazy and write with dry erase markers on your therapy table if it is the right surface. Students are shocked, and it makes it super easy to quickly provide them with a visual without needing tons of supplies.

You can use sentence starters or carrier phrases for many purposes. You can use them to help with recall of information. Sentence starters cue students to think about what they've learned and provide a framework for recalling and expressing that information. This structured approach reduces the cognitive load and makes recall more efficient.

For example, you can use prompts like "I remember that..." or "The main point was..." to guide students to focus on key information and retrieve it more easily. SLPs can also use this strategy to improve language comprehension. By providing a partial sentence, the SLP sets a clear expectation for the type of response, guiding students to think critically about what they read or heard and articulate their understanding in a coherent way.

When discussing a story or passage, you can use sentence starters to prompt students to express their understanding of the content. For example, you can provide the carrier phrases "This story is about..." or "The character felt... because...," which can help students focus on the main ideas and important details.

You can also use them to promote active listening and students' listening and engaging which each other's responses. You can provide a template for students to contribute meaningfully to discussions, thus enhancing comprehension and recall of the material discussed. For example, you can use sentence starters like "I agree with..." or "I noticed that...," which will encourage students to actively listen to their peers and engage in the conversation. These prompts help them connect their ideas with what others have said. Here are some more examples you can use:

- For summarizing: "The main point of this story is..."
- For predictions: "I think this will happen next because..."
- For inferences: "I can tell that the character feels... because..."

By consistently using sentence starters and carrier phrases, you can provide the necessary structure that can help your students better understand, recall, and express ideas effectively.

LEVERAGING AUDITORY CUES FOR SUCCESS

Many students struggle to process spoken information, especially when it's lengthy or complex. But for auditory learners, their natural strength lies in their ability to pick up on subtle details in what they hear. By teaching them to recognize and use auditory cues such as key phrases, changes in tone, and repeated ideas, you can help them unlock the meaning behind spoken language.

Think of these cues as guideposts on a trail: they point the way to important ideas, helping students navigate the content without getting lost. This strategy not only builds confidence but also equips them with skills to stay focused and organized, whether they're in a classroom discussion, watching a video, or listening to instructions.

This section explores how to explicitly teach students to identify and apply auditory cues to enhance their comprehension, all while building on their innate strengths as listeners. The goal is to make their ability to *hear* work smarter, not harder!

- **Introduce auditory cues:**
  - Explain that phrases like "the main reason," "for example," or changes in tone act as signals for important information.
  - Use an analogy: "These cues are like road signs—they guide you to what matters most."

- **Model the process (I do):**
  - Read a passage aloud, pausing at auditory cues.
  - Think aloud: "I heard 'the main idea is', so I'll focus on what comes next."
  - Highlight tone shifts or repetition as additional clues.

- **Practice together (we do):**
  - Listen to a passage together.
  - Stop after cues and ask the student: "What do you think this is pointing to?"
  - Provide prompts if needed: "What example follows 'for instance'?"

- **Independent practice (you do):**
  - Assign a short passage or audio clip.
  - Have the student identify key ideas using auditory cues and jot quick notes.
  - Encourage self-checking: "Why do you think this detail is important?"

Remember that not all students benefit from visual aids or visual strategies, but you need a tool for your toolbox for your auditory learners. It works because it builds on their natural auditory strengths, it simplifies spoken information by focusing on key phrases, and it encourages transferable listening skills for the classroom and beyond.

TAKING MULTISENSORY APPROACHES

Multisensory learning engages multiple senses (visual, auditory, kinesthetic, and tactile) to enhance comprehension and retention. This approach is particularly effective for students who struggle with traditional learning methods. These methods support memory, focus, and comprehension by activating multiple areas of the brain. The following sections outline some examples of multisensory approaches.

Tactile Tools

Use physical objects like blocks, counters, or cards to represent concepts. For example: Represent story elements (character, setting, problem, solution) with colored blocks, letting students rearrange them as they discuss the story.

For sentence-building, use puzzle pieces with parts of speech or phrases that students physically connect to form sentences.

Movement-Based Learning

Create activities where students physically move to match concepts. For example: Place key vocabulary words on the wall. Have students "run" to the correct word after hearing a definition or seeing a picture.

Auditory Tools

Record yourself or peers reading a passage. Have students listen while following along with a printed or visual version.

Use rhythm or music to teach concepts like syllable segmentation or sequencing (e.g., clapping out syllables or using songs to remember steps in a process).

SELF-ADVOCACY STRATEGIES: EMPOWERING STUDENTS TO ASK FOR WHAT THEY NEED

Teaching self-advocacy skills is one of the most impactful ways to support students' academic and social success. When students understand their needs and feel confident expressing them, they are more likely to engage actively and thrive in learning environments. This section discusses how to equip them with strategies to advocate for themselves when they need repetition, clarification, assistance, or any other type of support.

Understanding Their Needs

- **Recognize the signs**: Teach students to notice when they're confused, distracted, or unsure. They can ask themselves: "Did I understand that?" "Do I know what to do next?"
- **Reflect on triggers**: Help students identify situations that frequently cause difficulty, such as noisy environments, fast-paced instructions, or unfamiliar vocabulary.

Repetition Requests

- **What to say**: Practice phrases they can use to ask for repetition in a polite, specific way: "Could you please say that again more slowly?" and "Can you repeat the last part? I missed it."
- **Practice listening**: Encourage them to repeat key points after the second explanation to confirm understanding.

Clarification Strategies

- **Key phrases**: Equip students with simple, non-intimidating language to ask for clarification: "I'm not sure I understand. Could you explain it in a different way?" and "Can you give me an example of what you mean?"
- **Chunk the message**: Teach them to request smaller pieces of information: "Could you break that down into steps for me?" and "Can we go through one part at a time?"

Requesting Assistance

- **Prepare for advocacy**: Help students feel comfortable asking for help without fear of judgment: "I think I need some extra help with this part. Can we go over it together?" and "Can you show me how to get started?"
- **Role-playing**: Practice scenarios where they might need help—whether it's during group work, after class, or in a one-on-one meeting.

Managing Overwhelm

- **Pause and reflect**: Encourage students to ask for a moment to process: "Can I take a minute to think about that before I respond?" and "Can we take a quick break? I need to catch up."
- **Break it down**: Teach them to request a simpler explanation or fewer tasks: "This feels like a lot—can we focus on just one part right now?"

Building Confidence to Speak Up

- **Normalize advocacy**: Reinforce that asking for help or repetition is a strength, not a weakness.
- **Create scripts**: Provide go-to phrases for common situations, tailored to their specific needs.
- **Positive reinforcement**: Celebrate their efforts to advocate for themselves, even if they feel hesitant at first.

When to Seek Help Beyond the Classroom

- **Know the resources**: Educate students about who they can go to for support (e.g., teachers, counselors, or case managers).
- **Build a support network**: Encourage them to connect with peers or mentors who can help them navigate challenges.

Self-advocacy requires practice, so role-playing and modeling are essential. Create safe spaces for students to rehearse speaking up, experiment with phrasing, and reflect on what works best for them. Over time, these strategies will become second nature, empowering them to take control of their learning journey.

By helping students recognize their needs and giving them tools to address them, you're fostering independence, resilience, and confidence. These are skills that will serve them far beyond your therapy room.

SELF-ADVOCACY ROLE-PLAYING SCENARIOS

I know it can be a challenge to come up with role-playing scenarios on the spot. That's why this section includes a list of role-playing scenarios to help students practice self-advocacy in real-world contexts that you can use in your therapy room with your students. Role-playing scenarios allow students to practice self-advocacy in a safe, structured environment, building confidence and fluency in communicating their needs. This hands-on approach helps them prepare for real-world situations, fostering independence and problem-solving skills. These scenarios are designed to build their confidence and prepare them to request repetition, clarification, assistance, and accommodations effectively.

Requesting Repetition

- **Classroom instruction:** The teacher gives directions for an assignment, but the student didn't hear the last part. Practice asking the teacher to repeat the instructions.
- **Noisy environment:** During a group discussion in a loud cafeteria, the student misses what someone said. Practice politely asking for repetition.

Asking for Clarification

- **Ambiguous assignment:** The student is not sure how to format a homework assignment. Role-play how to ask the teacher for clarification.
- **Confusing instructions:** The teacher uses unfamiliar words while explaining a science experiment. Practice asking them to explain it differently.
- **Peer discussion:** A classmate explains their point in a group project, but it's unclear. Practice asking for clarification in a collaborative setting.

Requesting Assistance

- **Struggling with a concept:** The student doesn't understand a math problem. Practice how to ask the teacher for help after class.
- **Group work conflict:** The student is stuck on their part of a group project and needs help coordinating with teammates. Practice advocating for assistance.
- **Homework help:** The student is overwhelmed with a take-home assignment. Practice writing an email to their teacher asking for extra support.

Managing Overwhelm

- **Overloaded with tasks:** The student is given multiple assignments at once and doesn't know where to start. Practice asking the teacher to prioritize or extend a deadline.
- **In a fast-paced class:** The teacher moves through a lesson too quickly. Practice having the student raise their hand and ask for a slower explanation.

Handling Test Anxiety

- **Requesting extra time:** The student is struggling to finish a test. Practice asking for additional time if it's an accommodation they are entitled to.
- **Asking for a break:** The student is feeling overwhelmed during a test. Practice asking to take a short break to refocus.

Communicating Sensory Needs

- **Noisy classroom:** The student is distracted by noise in the classroom. Practice asking to move to a quieter spot.
- **Bright lighting:** The classroom lights are bothering the student. Practice asking for dimmer lighting or permission to wear a hat or sunglasses.

Advocating for Accommodations

- **Accessing notes:** The student missed part of the lesson and needs a copy of the teacher's notes. Practice asking politely.
- **Technology assistance:** The student struggles with handwriting and needs permission to use a laptop. Role-play how to explain why it helps.

Navigating Social Situations

- **Joining a conversation:** Peers are chatting, and the student wants to join but feels unsure how. Practice asking for clarification about what they're discussing and contributing.
- **Resolving a misunderstanding:** A classmate misinterprets something the student said. Practice clarifying their intent respectfully.

Dealing with Challenges at Work or Extracurriculars

- **Instructions at a job site:** The student's manager gives unclear instructions. Practice asking them to explain the task in more detail.
- **Sports or clubs:** The student is unsure how to complete their role in a team activity. Practice asking the coach or leader for guidance.

NOW WHAT?

Remember that you are trying to achieve quick wins. You want to see your students succeed and build their confidence. These are just some of the many possible strategies you can use to help students build on their strengths to overcome their weaknesses and teach skills differently so that they can grasp them. Not sure where to start? Start with their strengths. How can you build upon them and use one of these strategies to enhance them or overcome their weaknesses? What has been tried before? Why did it not work? The more you know about your students, the easier it will be to decide where to start with them.

When they finally grasp challenging tasks, it builds their confidence, gives them proof they can do such tasks, and gives them the encouragement to take on more challenges. They have experienced a quick win and enjoy the feeling of being successful. They will see how they can use these strategies in the classroom or outside of your therapy room.

You can share these approaches with their teachers to ensure carryover. Find what works best for your individual student. Just because they are working on a similar skill doesn't mean they will benefit from the same approaches.

Remember to explicitly teach all these strategies, model how to use them, and practice repeatedly. You cannot assume they will know how to use them, even if they were exposed to them previously. You need to take the time and show them how using these strategies will help them. If an approach doesn't work, don't be afraid to try something new.

As SLPs, we need to be okay with making mistakes and trying different things. We are scientists. We need to experiment. It doesn't make us a "bad SLP" for getting it wrong or not being completely certain where to start. It is trial and error. However, the more information you have about why a student has been struggling, what has been tried, and their learning styles, you can better determine where to start and do so confidently.

Steps for teaching skills:

1. Identify the student's strengths and challenges.
2. Choose a strategy that aligns with their needs.
3. Explicitly teach the strategy using "I do, we do, you do."
4. Practice repeatedly and adapt as needed.
5. Connect the strategy to classroom and real-life applications.

Hopefully, after reading this chapter, you have some new tools for your toolbox. You can always refer to this chapter when you need inspiration or reminders of ways to teach things differently. What new strategy will you try with your students?

CHAPTER 5

Connection over Data Collection

What if I told you the key to better student progress wasn't in your data binder but in how your students feel in your sessions? Let's be honest: we've all fantasized about tossing our data binder out the window. But before you do, let's talk about why it's okay to ease up on the tally marks and focus on what really matters—connection.

Data collection is so important in our practice that I felt like it needed a whole chapter. I discuss data more in Chapter 12, but I feel like I should discuss it here as well. You need data for Medicaid billing. You need data to determine how your students are progressing and for progress monitoring. We were taught in graduate school that we need to be constantly taking data. But is that the only approach? Taking tally marks the whole session can miss the point of the experience.

THAT OBSERVATION

I will never forget the day that I was once observed by an administrator. He sat in the back of the room. He did not make any facial expressions. He did not make eye contact with me. He just sat in the back and typed away on his laptop. What was he typing? Was it positive? Was it negative? The students were laughing at something I said, but he did not even make a flinch. I remember feeling so anxious, so self-conscious, so uncertain about my performance in that lesson. In that moment, I realized how we can come across as SLPs, taking data the entire session.

SLPs can appear authoritative and less approachable. If I felt anxious, even when confident in my lessons and ability to run my sessions, I can only imagine how my students feel when I am sitting there with my tally marks. I had to reflect, is this the only way to take data? To make my students feel anxious, worried about getting things wrong, wondering what I am constantly writing down?

Have you ever experienced this with an administrator? Maybe you remember your time in graduate school (or maybe you are in graduate school right now), and you recall having your supervisor constantly behind you, watching your every move, taking notes on your performance. How did it make you feel? Were you comfortable? How would you describe this experience? Take a moment and reflect on how you feel about taking tests, working under pressure, or just being observed. Maybe you recall your heart racing, overthinking, or second guessing your actions.

VIEWING IT FROM THEIR PERSPECTIVE

We need to consider how our students feel when we are taking data or in trials mode (i.e., busy trying to get enough trials in and not noticing how our students are doing, why they might be getting something wrong, or what is even causing them to get things right). Do we want our students feeling that way all the time with us and viewing our sessions as high intensity and stressful?

Take a moment to think about your last session. How much time did you spend teaching versus tallying? How did it make you feel? How did your students respond? Did you get the data you were hoping for? I will never forget when I decided to try something new for the first time. One of my students rarely participated. But when I stopped taking data for an entire session and just chatted about his favorite basketball team, everything changed. The next week, he was eager to try, and I saw progress like never before. It doesn't always take much to get a huge return.

When we spend the entire session taking data, we are spending the session testing. More tally marks don't mean a better session. We need to take the time to teach. That is why students are there with us. We need to be mindful of this when we work with them.

TEACHING, NOT TESTING

If you spend your days just taking data, you could miss opportunities to teach and to notice what strategies your students respond well to. If you are focusing on getting a specific number of trials in, you may be missing what your students truly need in order to learn the skill. More trials don't mean better results if they have not learned it properly. Taking tally marks during a session can feel like playing Tetris—except you're trying to fit your data into tiny boxes while also juggling 5,000 other things. And no one is cheering when you clear a row.

You are probably wondering, "Okay, great, but I need data." Maybe consider putting it on the shelf for some of the session. Maybe even for an entire session.

Take the time to introduce concepts, teach the skills, reflect on what strategies are working, and practice them to build confidence. You can take a few moments at the end of a session to collect some data to monitor progress. One trial is data. One opportunity to show if they grasp a concept—that's data. Especially with longer passages, your students may only have one opportunity to demonstrate a skill fully in a session. If a student is struggling to learn a new skill, they may need a new strategy introduced, or they may need more opportunities to view models. They may never get to do a skill completely independently during that session. That is okay.

When it comes to data, I find the anecdotal data is more essential than the tally marks or trials. On a sticky note, jot down one anecdotal observation you've made recently about a student. How could this guide your next session? Some things to consider documenting:

- What strategy worked? What did not work?
- What length was the text?
- Did they have choices or not?
- How many models or repetitions were needed?
- Were they independent or needed assistance?
- What other observations did you make?

This approach can help you more when it comes to planning the next session or if you need to back up and work on more fundamental skills.

When the Administrator Insists on Hard Data

There are administrators that want data for their own purposes. They may need it to show for funding, hiring, or just staff evaluations. You need to be an advocate for your students and their needs. You can educate administrators on the benefits of not taking data the entire session. Promise them you will have data, just not for every second of the session. It doesn't mean the session didn't happen. You can share with them that the math teacher only assesses at the end of the unit. That doesn't mean teaching didn't happen. Students need to learn the math concepts in order to do well on the assessment. The same goes for SLPs.

When You Miss Something Critical

We are busy and have a lot to remember. We cannot remember everything and data helps us. You can jot down the anecdotal data too. But tally mark after tally mark isn't going to help you remember more. It will keep you feeling busy, but it will be harder to focus on the students in front of you that need your attention, need to trust you, and need to know that you care.

Thoughts from the Field

I asked my SLP Elevate member, Elsha Young, about her thoughts on data collection and building rapport. She currently works as a virtual SLP with students in Alaska. She reported, "And sometimes data doesn't happen. It's okay. Doesn't have to, doesn't need to most of the time. I have life skills, kids. They're that. I listen. I just listen. Nine times out of 10, they have something more important that they need to talk about that day. And so I listen. How are you doing today? How are your classes going? What's going on in your life? Oh, grandma's in the hospital again? Okay, let's talk about that. A lot of times I will pull up a video and it's one of the YouTube cheat sheets. I'll pull that up and say, hey, which one of these do you want to watch today? Let's watch a video together. And that's how I've gotten a lot of engagement is I let them choose. I give them choices, I've built rapport. They trust that I will listen."

Elsha has realized it is more about trust than data. When students trust us, they will work with us and that is when the progress can occur. If they don't trust us, you are spending your time trying to pull data out of them. You will get frustrated. They will get frustrated. What is more important?

Let's discuss a sample format of a session and discuss when data could fit in. When planning for a session, I like to consider and incorporate the following:

- **IEP goal:** What is the goal that you are addressing?
- **Session objective:** What is the objective for this specific session that will help the student get to the annual goal by the end of the year? Where are they currently at? What specific skill or strategy are you teaching or practicing in this session?
- **Introduction:** How are you introducing the topic? How is it relevant to them? When might they have heard this concept before?
- **Strategy:** How are you teaching the strategy to them? How are you teaching it to them, so they grasp it? Are you utilizing graphic organizers, note-taking, sorting answers into categories, and so on?
- **Materials:** What materials do you need to complete the lesson?
- **Conclusion:** How are you wrapping up the lesson so they understand the strategy and how they can use it outside of the speech room?
- **Data collection/assessment:** How are you determining performance? How are you assessing if they learned the new skill or made progress while practicing?

Here's a completed sample:

- **IEP goal:** Student will verbally express main ideas of passages heard.
- **Session objective:** Student will verbally express main ideas of fictional paragraphs heard.
- **Introduction:** Has your teacher ever asked you "what is it all about?" after reading a story? How did you respond? It can be hard to know exactly what to say or how much to say. I am going to show you a way to answer so you know exactly what to do when that question comes up. You only need one sentence! It will show your teachers that you understand what was read.
- **Strategy:** Visual showing main idea = "who?" "what happened?"
- **Materials:** Main idea visual, task card game to practice expressing main ideas using fictional paragraph stories.
- **Conclusion:** So when you hear the question "what is it all about?" Do you need one sentence or many sentences? What do you need to say that will show your teachers that you understand?
- **Data collection/assessment:** After the SLP models how they use the visual and thinks about her responses, student will have the opportunity to practice using the SLP model. Then, they will play the task card game, taking turns listening to a paragraph and expressing the main idea. The SLP will note how many were correct versus incorrect, if they used the visual, if they struggled with "who" or "what happened," or if they had a hard time attending to the paragraph heard.

As you can see from this example, you need to take the time teach. You need to take the opportunity to practice. Then, once students grasp it, you can collect data on their performance. The teaching is the important part, not the data. As you may have also noted, I indicated what informal or anecdotal data I plan to collect. What are things I want to make sure that I observe? That information will be extremely helpful as I plan the follow-up session. Do you need to go backward and work on listening for significant details? Do you need more chunking of the paragraph and go sentence by sentence? Do they recognize when they need auditory information repeated? If they got things wrong, what did they do instead?

When you have large caseloads, the more you can document the better. It can be hard to remember everything that happened throughout the day with each individual student. That is the benefit of collecting data and documenting that anecdotal information. You may not remember once that next group comes in and distracts you. You may not remember which strategy was tried and which was effective.

When it comes to data collection systems, there is no right or wrong way. As with a lot of things in this field, it is personal preference and what works best for you. Some SLPs prefer sticky notes; some even take data on a piece of tape and transfer it over.

Here's a rundown of a method I find helpful:

- I take data for a group on a sheet for the day. I laminate a group data form, put it on a clipboard, write with dry erase all day, and transfer the data into a data binder at the end of the day when I am reflecting on the day and making my plans for the next sessions.
- Once the information is transferred, I erase the laminated sheet and start fresh the next day.
- My data binder contains tabs for each student. Each student has a section in a large binder with their goals, an attendance form, and a sheet to document progress over time. Of course, I have space on that sheet for anecdotal data.

> **TIP**
>
> You can get access to all my printable data forms for free, along with all of my other book resources at www.speechtimefun.com/book.

Some SLPs prefer the digital route, going paperless, and seeing progress on a screen. There are many tools out there, but I custom created one that is included in my SLP Elevate membership. It allows members to create student profiles with all important information and take data individually or as a group. You can enter data manually at the end of a session or day or you can use the tracker and mark + or – how they are doing in the moment. Of course, it has a space to note anecdotal data. You can view student reports, print them out, and even download charts to include in reports. It is just another option for data collection.

It doesn't matter what system you use, as long as you are able to take the time to teach the skills, incorporate data other than tally marks, and reflect on what worked and what didn't. Just like anything, you can always change your system and try something new.

Data Collection Alternatives

There are methods to data collection other than tally marks. Incorporating data alternatives can empower SLPs to track student progress more holistically and flexibly, while still fulfilling professional and billing requirements. The following sections dive deeper into specific alternatives and practical strategies.

Anecdotal Data Logs

Instead of focusing solely on tally marks, use anecdotal logs to capture richer details about each session.

What to document:

- Observations about student behavior, engagement, or mood (e.g., "Student seemed distracted during longer passages.")
- Specific strategies used and their effectiveness (e.g., "Used sentence starters; student became more independent after two trials.")
- Environmental or contextual factors (e.g., "Group dynamic seemed to encourage participation today.")

How to track:

- Use a notebook, a digital app, or sticky notes.
- Develop a shorthand system for quick, consistent notes (e.g., "+" for progress, "–" for struggles, "?" for uncertainties).

Student Self-Assessments

Give students the opportunity to reflect on their performance. Why it works:

- Encourages metacognition and self-regulation
- Provides insight into their perspective and areas they find challenging
- How to implement it:
- Create a simple scale (e.g., "How well do you think you did on this activity?" 1–5).
- Use visual aids, such as emoji charts, for younger students.
- Incorporate reflective prompts, such as "What felt easy or hard today?" and "What strategy helped you the most?"

Peer Feedback

If you're working in group settings, incorporate peer observations and feedback. Example activity: After a group practice session, ask peers to share:

- What did you notice about how your classmate answered?
- What strategy seemed to help them the most?

Benefits:

- Encourages collaboration and listening skills
- Allows students to reflect on their peers' progress, which can reinforce their own learning

Rubrics and Checklists

Design simple rubrics or checklists for common IEP goals and skills. Why it works:

- Provides consistency in how performance is measured across sessions
- Reduces reliance on tally marks while still offering structured data

How to implement it:

- Create rubrics with categories like independence level (e.g., fully independent, prompt needed, verbal model required).
- Use checklists to track progress over time (e.g., "Successfully answered main idea questions in 3 out of 5 trials.").

Parent and Teacher Input

Incorporate insights from those who see the student outside of sessions. How to collect this data:

- Use a brief questionnaire or form for parents/teachers to note observations (e.g., "Has the student used any new vocabulary at home?").
- Schedule periodic check-ins to gather qualitative data on generalization of skills.

Incorporating these alternatives allows you to collect meaningful data while maintaining a focus on teaching and building connections. These methods can reduce stress for both you and your students, making sessions more productive and enjoyable.

DATA IS IMPORTANT

Data collection is necessary. It is important. We need it for billing and to make recommendations. We may be asked to present it to defend a case. I don't want you walking away from this chapter saying that I told you not to collect data. I am just saying to not let data become your only focus. Don't let it control you. Your students are there to learn. You need to teach and give them opportunities to learn. You also want them feeling safe to make mistakes. If you want your students to work and take risks, you need them feeling safe with you.

That is why starting with those quick wins is so essential. You want your students trusting you, believing in themselves, and seeing how your instruction will help them outside of your speech room. You want learning to be fun, even if you aren't playing a game. If you are always testing, that isn't fun. If you are constantly writing everything down, you are not paying attention to them and making the connections necessary to build trust.

NOW WHAT?

Will you put your data binder away? Will you start taking more anecdotal data? How will you view data differently since reading this chapter? I challenge you to put the binder down for a session or two and see what happens when you prioritize connection and teaching over constant data collection.

Here is a quick checklist of ideas to try when it comes to data collection:

- Take five minutes of every session to observe and connect.
- Write down one anecdotal observation per student.
- Use a visual or strategy instead of a tally sheet for at least one activity.

Whether you pick one or try them all, try something new and see if you get a new result! I would love to hear how it goes! Feel free to share pictures with me on Instagram and tag me. You're not just teaching skills; you're shaping confidence, trust, and independence. When you focus on connection over collection, you give your students a reason to keep showing up—and that's data you can't measure with tally marks.

Creative Competence

In this section, which includes Chapters 6 through 8, you learn ways to incorporate some creativity into your sessions to keep them motivating and fun. Now that you have a better understanding of what to work on and how to work on it to get quick wins and build momentum, you need to keep the momentum going as you challenge your students. You want your students to want to come to speech! This section discusses how to achieve that goal. Ready to be the fun SLP? Let's go!

CHAPTER 6

The Importance of Incorporating Student Interests and Goals

I remember applying to graduate school. It felt like a scavenger hunt created by a very determined villain: gather recommendations, write essays, fill out endless applications. . . all while hoping you'd somehow survive the GRE without crying in the test center bathroom (again). There was so much to do, things that were new to me, yet I still did it. I was motivated. I wanted to pursue this career. I saw the benefit of pushing through the challenging tasks. What motivated you to push through your own challenges, whether in graduate school or your professional career? How might that relate to what your students need to feel motivated in speech therapy? Just like we needed to be motivated by our own challenging tasks to complete them and not give up, our students need to be motivated to be willing to participate in challenging tasks.

I'll never forget the day one of my students flat out asked me, "Why do I have to come to speech? It's not like it's going to help me." I froze. In that moment, I realized two things: One, this student hadn't bought in. Two, I hadn't shown them how what we were doing could help them in their real life.

Your students each have their own perspectives and experiences when it comes to their learning, communication, and difficulties. Learning is hard for them. They may have a negative view of school, and even speech. They have been receiving speech for years and are tired of it, embarrassed by it, and very aware of their learning and communication difficulties. They need to see the value—because let's be honest, if you asked any teenager whether they'd rather stay in class or come to speech, they're going to pick "neither." They need to understand why they must leave class to come to the speech room. They don't want to do arbitrary activities. They need to believe in the process.

INTRODUCING CREATIVE COMPETENCE

Since most secondary students have negative views on learning and going to speech, and they are more aware of their learning and communications difficulties, you need to approach working with this age group differently than working with the younger elementary students. Secondary students are more complex, requiring an approach to sessions that I call creative competence.

What does creative competence mean in practice? It's about combining adaptability, creativity, and a deep understanding of each student's needs. Here's how you can break it down:

1. Understand your students:

   - Take the time to truly learn about your students. Use casual conversations, observations, and interest inventories to uncover what makes them tick.
   - Think beyond surface-level likes—dig into what motivates them, what they value, and their personal goals. For example, does your student want to improve communication skills to ask a crush to prom or to get through a group project without anxiety?

2. Incorporate their interests:

   - Once you know their hobbies, passions, and even quirks, find ways to tie them into your sessions.
   - For example, if your student loves sports, use game commentaries to practice summarizing, or create scenarios where they're a coach giving instructions (targeting sequencing or clarity).

3. Make connections to real life:

   - Show students how what you're working on in speech directly applies to their lives. This could be preparing for job interviews, explaining ideas in a classroom setting, or even communicating better with family or friends.
   - For example: "This strategy we're practicing will help you in job interviews when you need to explain your past experiences clearly and confidently."

When you implement creative competence, you're showing students that speech isn't just another pull-out class—it's something that directly improves their ability to reach their goals and enjoy the things they love. How well do you currently know your students' interests and goals? What's one thing you could do tomorrow to learn more about them?

You cannot spend the entire year fighting with students to come to speech. And you don't likely have the luxury of small caseloads to spend all your time trying to craft creative ways to trick them into coming to speech. You cannot be running around buildings chasing them down when they try to avoid coming to speech. Wouldn't it be more enjoyable to go to work every day having students run down the hall to come to see you versus running the other way each time you approach them?

WHY THEIR INTERESTS ARE YOUR SECRET WEAPON

By incorporating interests and goals, you can plan lessons that are engaging enough to keep them from counting ceiling tiles or asking, "When can I leave?" every five minutes. Think of one student you have who struggles to engage in sessions. How might incorporating their interests make a difference in their motivation and progress? You can easily show them how what you are doing will help them in the classroom and in their everyday life. This will also allow you to plan quickly and easily around themes and concepts.

This section explains how to gather student interests and goals, how to find resources, and even how to tweak lessons you are already doing to be able to demonstrate to your students how what you are doing is relevant to them. You do not need a million materials or tons of time. You don't need a completely unique lesson for each group. You just need an open mind and the ability to see the value.

Sample Conversation Starters to Learn Students' Interests

Building rapport and understanding students' interests and personal goals is crucial for creating meaningful and engaging therapy sessions. These sample conversation starters are designed to be open-ended, low-pressure, and adaptable to your students' comfort levels. Use these prompts to spark conversations and learn more about their world.

General Interests

- What's your favorite thing to do when you're not in school?
- If you could spend an entire weekend doing just one thing, what would it be?
- What's something you've always wanted to try but haven't yet?
- What's the last thing you watched on YouTube or Netflix? Did you like it?
- What's your favorite app or game right now?

Hobbies and Activities

- Do you play any sports or wish you could? Which ones?
- Do you have any hobbies, like drawing, playing video games, or making music?
- If you could learn any new skill or hobby, what would it be?
- What's the most fun thing you did this past month?
- Do you like working on projects, like building or creating things? What's something cool you've made before?

Pop Culture and Entertainment

- Who's your favorite singer, band, or music artist?
- What's your favorite TV show, movie, or series? Why do you like it?
- If you could be any character from a video game or movie, who would you pick and why?
- Do you follow any YouTubers, TikTok-ers, or streamers? Who's your favorite?
- What's the coolest thing you've seen on social media lately?

Aspirations

- What's something you're really good at or want to get better at?
- What do you think you might want to do after high school?
- Do you have any big dreams or goals for the future?
- What's one thing you'd like to accomplish this school year?
- If you could have any job in the world, what would it be?

Favorites and Preferences

- What's your favorite food or snack? Do you like to cook or bake?
- What's your favorite holiday or time of year? Why?
- Do you have a favorite animal or pet? If you could have any pet, what would it be?
- What's your favorite subject in school—or the least boring one?
- What's the best trip or vacation you've ever been on?

Social and Relational Topics

- Who do you usually hang out with at school? What do you like to do together?
- If you could plan a perfect day with your friends, what would you do?
- What's something you and your family like to do together?

- Do you prefer spending time with people, or do you like some quiet time too?
- What's something funny that's happened to you or your friends recently?

Personal Insights

- What's something people don't know about you that you think is really cool?
- What's one thing that always makes you happy?
- If you could change one rule at school or at home, what would it be?
- What's something you've worked really hard on and felt proud of?
- Do you like working with other people or by yourself? Why?

These conversation starters can be used as icebreakers, in one-on-one discussions, or as part of group activities. They help you connect with your students, learn their interests, and show them that you care about what matters to them. Over time, these discussions will naturally build trust and lead to more engaging and personalized therapy sessions.

You should also be participating and sharing answers to the questions as well. Let your students get to know you. You don't need to share all of your deep dark secrets or your home address but let them in a little bit. If you want them to trust you, they need to feel like they know you. They may also find fun in learning that they have similar interests as you! Show them that you aren't just a "teacher," but a real person.

Sample Conversation Starters to Learn Students' Personal and Academic Goals

Understanding your students' personal and academic goals is essential for designing therapy sessions that feel meaningful and aligned with their aspirations. These conversation starters help you gain insight into what matters most to your students and how you can connect their goals to your therapy work.

Exploring Personal Goals

- What's something you've always wanted to achieve but haven't had the chance yet?
- If you could learn any new skill, what would it be?
- What's one thing you'd love to accomplish outside of school this year?
- Do you have any personal goals, like getting a driver's license, starting a job, or joining a club?
- What's something that would make you feel really proud of yourself?

Discussing Academic Goals

- Is there a specific subject you'd like to get better at this year?
- What's something you'd like to improve on in school—like studying, writing, or participating in class?
- Do you have any big school-related goals, like making honor roll or passing a certain class?
- What's one thing you'd like to change about how you approach schoolwork?
- Do you have a goal for after high school, like college, a trade, or a job? What steps do you think you need to take to get there?

Combining Personal and Academic Aspirations

- What's something you're learning in school that you think could help you in your life outside of school?
- How do you think doing well in school can help you reach your personal dreams?
- Do you feel like there's anything standing in the way of your goals? How can we work on that together?
- If you could pick one thing to focus on improving this year, what would it be—inside or outside of school?
- Is there a project, assignment, or activity coming up that you're excited about—or nervous about?

Identifying Strengths and Challenges

- What's one thing you're really good at that you'd like to get even better at?
- Is there something you've been struggling with in school or life that you'd like to work on?
- Do you feel more confident about certain skills or subjects than others? What are they?
- What's one challenge you've faced recently, and how did you handle it?
- If you could have help with one thing in school, what would it be?

Tapping Into Aspirations

- What do you hope to be doing five years from now? Ten years from now?
- Is there a job or career that sounds interesting to you? Why?
- Do you think the things we're working on here can help you in your future? How?
- What's one thing you'd love to do after you graduate high school?
- If you could create your dream future, what would it look like?

Making Therapy Relevant

- How do you think improving your communication skills can help you in school or life?
- What's something you wish you felt more confident doing in or out of school?
- Are there any specific skills or topics you'd like to work on in our sessions?
- What's one area where you'd like to feel more successful?
- How can I help you work toward your goals—both personal and academic?

These prompts will help you start meaningful conversations with your students about their aspirations. Over time, these discussions can help you tailor your therapy sessions to address their goals and show them how your work together aligns with their vision for the future. You may be surprised by your students' responses!

Let's Talk Examples

This section shares some practical examples to help you see what I mean. Consider these approaches to incorporating your students' interests and desires into your session activities.

Interest-Based Lessons

For students who loves sports:

- Use sports articles or play-by-play commentary to work on sequencing, vocabulary, or summarizing.
- For articulation goals, have them "announce" plays using their target sounds.

  For students who are into video games:

- Analyze character motivations and storylines from their favorite games to target inferencing and predicting.
- Use gaming terminology to work on vocabulary or sentence formulation.

Goal-Oriented Lessons

For students who want a job:

- Practice mock interviews to build confidence and conversational skills.
- Work on functional language like following multistep directions or asking clarifying questions.

For students applying to college:

- Use college applications or scholarship essays to practice organizing thoughts, using complex sentences, or editing for grammar.

You Tried and It Didn't Work

You asked about their interests, and they gave you a blank stare. You planned a whole lesson about Fortnite, and suddenly they don't "really like it anymore." Welcome to the wonderful world of working with teenagers! Before you give up on the idea entirely, troubleshoot what might have gone wrong and explore ways to refine your approach.

They Won't Share Their Interests

Some students are naturally guarded or unsure how to answer when asked directly about their interests. Instead of asking, "What do you like?" try more creative, low-pressure ways to uncover their likes:

- **Observe them:** What are they wearing? Are they doodling on their notebooks? Do they have stickers on their water bottles? These can give you clues about their hobbies or personality.
- **Ask indirect questions:** Instead of "What's your favorite hobby?" try "What's the last movie or show you watched?" or "If you could spend the weekend doing anything, what would it be?"
- **Explore together:** Offer a list of possibilities and let them choose. For example: "Do you prefer sports, music, video games, or something else?" This helps students who may not know how to articulate their interests.

Their Interests Didn't Translate to Engagement

Sometimes, students might be interested in a topic, but the activity doesn't connect for them. Reflect on these key factors:

- **Were the materials appropriate?** Check if the reading level, length, or complexity of the material matched their ability. If a passage is too hard (or too easy), they'll disengage quickly.
- **Was the activity clear and relevant?** Ensure the connection between the activity and their interests was explicit. For example, don't just use a sports

article—explain how summarizing it helps them communicate better with teammates or coaches.

- **Did they have the right tools?** Did you scaffold the lesson with strategies or supports (e.g., graphic organizers or sentence starters)? Students may need these tools to feel confident tackling the task.

They Still Don't Respond

If your efforts still didn't click, don't write off this approach—try reframing how you introduce it. For instance:

- **Use curiosity:** If they don't want to talk about themselves, ask them to teach *you* about something they're interested in. For example: "I don't know much about video games—what's the most exciting part of the game you're playing?" This flips the dynamic and puts them in control, which can spark engagement.
- **Try a tangential approach:** Sometimes, the interest itself might not align directly with a speech goal. Instead, use it as a conversation starter or warm-up before transitioning to the main task.

Why Troubleshooting Is Worth It

When students don't respond immediately, it's not a sign that this approach doesn't work—it's a signal to tweak your methods. Go back to the strategies in earlier chapters: Are the goals realistic? Are the lessons scaffolded? Are you setting them up for quick wins to build confidence?

Finding the right balance takes time, but once students see how speech connects to their interests and goals, their engagement and motivation can transform. Keep experimenting until you find what resonates!

If your goal is to have more fun and interactive lessons that have students excited to come to speech, this is the ultimate way to get that accomplished. You can still be effective without doing this. Without their buy-in, you'll end up spending sessions talking to the wall—or worse, watching them perfect their "I'm-ignoring-you" look. Spoiler: They're good at it.

You want your students to progress and ultimately no longer need you. You don't want them receiving speech and language services forever and be pulled out of class forever. Help them achieve their goal of no longer needing the service by showing them they can learn and have fun at the same time.

FUN VERSUS GAMES: STRIKING THE RIGHT BALANCE

Let's talk about fun and games in speech therapy. It's a topic that often sparks debate: Do we need to play games every session? Absolutely not. Should we avoid games altogether because teenagers are "too old" for them? Also, no. (Remember, this is the same age group that can spend hours arguing over the best Dorito flavor, so let's not assume they're too cool for everything.)

Here's the thing—learning is hard for your students. They're tackling tough skills, often with a history of struggle or failure, and you need to create an environment where they feel safe, supported, and maybe even excited to try. Fun doesn't always mean games, but it does mean engagement. If you can make learning enjoyable, you've won half the battle.

Games have their place in speech therapy, even for adolescents, but they're a tool—not the goal. A well-timed game can:

- **Break the ice:** Perfect for new groups or when students are feeling particularly resistant.
- **Lower the stakes:** Games create a low-pressure way to practice skills, reducing anxiety around "getting it right."
- **Encourage natural language use:** Many games require communication, collaboration, and quick thinking—all great ways to target goals in an organic way.
- **Build motivation:** Sometimes, the promise of a game can keep students engaged through more challenging parts of the session.

That said, not every session needs to include a game. Fun can also come from:

- Creative, interest-based lessons tied to student goals
- Collaborative projects where students work together to solve problems
- Dynamic discussions on topics they care about

If you're worried that games might feel "babyish" to older students, remember this: It's all in how you present them. Use age-appropriate games and themes that align with their interests. For example:

- Instead of Candy Land, try trivia games like Jeopardy with topics they choose.
- Replace preschool board games with interactive, competitive activities like escape room challenges or scavenger hunts.
- Incorporate digital tools like Kahoot or Blooket for a modern twist that feels more relevant to their world.

If you have a student who rolls their eyes at the mere mention of a game? No problem—fun can come from other strategies, like role-playing real-world scenarios or debating pop culture topics.

Now, let's address the flipside. If you play games every session, students might start seeing speech therapy as playtime instead of a space to build real skills. The key is balance:

- **Set clear expectations:** Before introducing a game, explain how it connects to their goals. Example: "We're playing this word association game to practice quick thinking and building connections between ideas—skills you'll need for class discussions."
- **Mix it up:** Alternate between games, structured lessons, and collaborative activities to keep students guessing and engaged.
- **Keep control:** If students constantly ask, "Are we playing a game today?" try redirecting their focus.

TIP

Hang a sign with reminders like, "Speech is for learning, not just for games." (Grab my free printable sign at https://www.teacherspayteachers .com/Product/Things-We-Do-Not-Say-In-Speech-Signs-FREEBIE- 3917177?st=58cb322780448a91dfb0ca431ddd80db.)

Fun is essential in speech therapy—not because it's entertaining, but because it builds a foundation of trust and engagement. Whether it's through a game, a project, or an interest-driven lesson, creating an enjoyable environment encourages students to take risks, make mistakes, and ultimately learn. So, while every session doesn't need to end with a game, every session should have a moment where your students feel connected, engaged, and successful.

How do you currently balance fun and productivity in your sessions? What's one way you could add more engagement—whether through games, projects, or interest-based lessons—while staying focused on goals?

YOUR QUICK START GUIDE TO CREATIVE COMPETENCE

Here is a checklist for incorporating interests and goals:

- **Step 1:** Ask about their interests or observe.
- **Step 2:** Identify a goal or skill they're working on.
- **Step 3:** Brainstorm one activity that ties their interest to the goal.
- **Step 4:** Make it actionable (e.g., find a short article, prepare a prompt).
- **Step 5:** Reflect afterward: Did it work? What could you tweak next time?

NOW WHAT?

Hopefully you are starting to see the value and benefits of incorporating interests and goals into your speech sessions. If you want your students participating, you need to give them a reason.

Take a moment to reflect on your best and worst sessions—the ones where you nailed it and the ones where you felt like your student deserved a gold medal for avoidance tactics. What worked? What didn't? And what might you tweak next time to turn "meh" into "wow, that was fun!" If you are new to the field and have yet to have failed or successful sessions, maybe ask your mentor or supervisor. What did they learn from their successful and failed sessions? Ask them about their feelings about games in speech. Learn from others. Listen to all perspectives. The more we know, the more we can learn.

The next chapter dives into creative ways to gather information about your students' interests and goals—because sometimes, the best ideas come from the most unexpected places!

CHAPTER 7

Building Rapport

Rapport. We hear that word often but what does it really mean? And why is it so essential for SLPs, but more importantly for SLPs working with secondary students? According to the dictionary, "rapport" means "a close and harmonious relationship in which the people or groups concerned understand each other's feelings or ideas and communicate well." Notice the word "communicate" is in there. If you want your students to communicate and participate in speech sessions, they need to know you understand them. They also need to understand you.

Rapport is particularly vital for secondary students. Teenagers are at a developmental stage where trust, autonomy, and social connections are critical. Many secondary students have a history of academic struggles, making them more resistant or cautious in new environments.

Building rapport creates a safe space for risk-taking, which is essential for communication growth.

MORE THAN A RING

I will never forget my first year working in a high school. I was in my early 20s, only 5 feet tall, and completely clueless on my role with this age group. I did not know the curriculum or even why they had the goals they had. Do I just use curriculum? Where do I find materials to teach these things? I was not an ELA teacher, but all I could find were worksheets in ELA workbooks. My students did not want to be there, and they had no problem letting me know it. They probably also noticed the scared look on my face daily. It didn't help that I was constantly mistaken as a student and asked for a hall pass. I was only in that building for a few periods a day, and no one knew who I was. I was also the only SLP in the building.

These students were going to walk all over me. I had to do something. That was when I noticed one of the senior girls in the group looking at my new engagement ring. "Yes. I just got engaged," I told her. Her eyes lit up. That was when I stopped my boring lesson and just let her and the other students ask me questions. They were curious and wanted to know more about me. I didn't need to tell them all my deep dark secrets, but I let them know more about the person working with them on difficult tasks they did not want to work on. They were excited to learn more. I saw a shift in the way they came to the following session. I told them if they did the work we needed to accomplish, in the last few minutes they could ask me anything again. They worked. I even let them draw on the Smart Board the room had for the last few minutes of the session. Of course, that one senior girl drew engagement rings on the Smart Board. She was having fun. She wanted to do the work for me.

I realized in that moment that learning is hard for these students. If we want them to work for us and do difficult things, they need to trust us. They need to want to work with us. If we rush and jump into working on goals and do not take the time to get to know them and let them get to know us, they will never be fully motivated with us. I get it we need to work on goals and have to document them for billing purposes. But our students are more important. That is why we are there—for their well-being, their progress. We need them to trust us. They are going to make mistakes with us, take risks with us, and even ask us for help. They need to know we won't judge them and that we are there to help them. If a new administrator came to observe you and you didn't know them or trust them, how would you feel if you made a mistake in your session?

In case you were wondering about that high school senior: Strangely enough, years later, a mother of a student of mine came up to me and asked me if I once worked in a different school district. I told her that in fact I did. She was that student. Once she told me who she was I immediately recalled her and her interest in asking me about my engagement and wedding plans. Luckily, at this point in my career, I knew the importance of rapport, and her daughter had already built that with me!

A few years ago, I was taking my daughter to the pediatrician. While there, I heard a familiar voice in another room. I don't live in the same neighborhood that I work in, so I didn't expect it to be a current or previous student. But sure enough, when we were leaving, I saw that it was in fact a student I had five years prior. He was a challenging student and was especially difficult because I was pregnant with my first at the time. He would often take off while I was transitioning him from his classroom to my speech room. I would have to call down to the security guard at the other end of the hallway to help since I couldn't run so fast while pregnant.

Anyway, when I saw this student, he looked at me and said, "Hi, Miss Speech." At first I was shocked he recognized me and even remembered my "name." But after reflecting for a moment, I wasn't surprised. I had made a connection with this student. I had an impact. All of that hard work and all the stressful moments were worth it.

Rapport is more than just doing icebreakers in the beginning of the year. It is important to get the conversation started, but rapport goes beyond that. If rapport was just about icebreakers, we'd all be professionals by now. You need them to know that you care. When you take the time to build that relationship, anything is possible! Your students may even seek you out and stop by your room to tell you something when it isn't even their time for speech. I once had a student who would ask his teacher to go to the bathroom and take the "long way" to stop by my room to say hello. He would just pop right in, sit down, and want to make small talk. I prefer that over them running away from me when they see me in the hallway!

COMFORT CONTRACT

Students come from different backgrounds and experiences when it comes to learning and communication. Do they have an experience of being bullied because of their speech? Do they hate to get attention from the teacher because they don't know the answers in class? What about their experiences of getting things wrong in the past? Have kids laughed at them in the past? Let's talk about past speech experiences. Maybe they have a history of working on the same goal over and over and not seeing progress. Maybe they are frustrated with constantly working on the same articulation sound or even language comprehension goal.

You need to be always mindful that you might not know students' past experiences. You need to be striving to make them feel safe with you. That is why I like to generate a comfort contract with my students. I like to have a dialogue with them at the beginning of the year and remind them throughout about the appropriate behavior and expectations in my speech room. What should they do if they need help? They need to know that I am there for them and not there to embarrass them if something is challenging or if they get something wrong. I am there to teach them, not test them. Here are some example statements you can include in a comfort contract:

- "I will be patient with myself and others."
- "I will celebrate mistakes as part of learning."

Students also need to trust their peers in the group. They need to understand that they all have different strengths and weaknesses and that they can all learn from each other. This also goes back to the different learning styles and understanding that, although they may all be different, they can all still learn and grow. They should know what is expected of them in the group when others are responding. How should they behave if a peer gets something wrong, needs more support, or needs more time to accomplish a task?

The more you have these conversations, build these routines and expectations, and hold them all accountable, the more they will trust you and the more they will trust each other. This is why I love group therapy. Once they realize they can learn from each other and that they are not alone in needing help, they can rely on each other and have a lot of fun.

Have your students generate a list of what would make them feel safe and comfortable in your speech room. To help facilitate the contract discussion, use sentence starters or prompts:

- What makes you feel safe to try new things?
- How should we handle it if someone gets something wrong?

Let them discuss with each other how they want to be respected. Generate a list and have them all agree upon it and even sign it. Refer to this list if anything comes up that goes against this contract. They wrote it. Remind them of the benefits of sticking to it.

SAMPLE RAPPORT-BUILDING ACTIVITIES

I like to incorporate some simple activities at the beginning of the year to remind my students that everyone has different strengths and weaknesses, everyone makes mistakes, and everyone overcomes challenges. These activities highlight the benefits of not giving up. You can do these throughout the year as well. If you are wondering how speech goals tie into these activities, by the end of this book you will realize you can take any activity and target a goal with it. But to be able to work on a goal, you need your students to be willing to take risks. You need them to feel comfortable. Sometimes, it is okay to just say progress on a goal is zero for the day.

Strengths Strand

Have you ever taken strands of paper, made loops, and looped them together? I like to give my students pieces of paper and let them write down one thing they are good at. What is their strength? What can they teach the group? Here are some prompts to help students identify their strengths:

- What's something you're good at that your friends ask you for help with?
- What's something you enjoy doing that you feel proud of?

Encourage students to share how they developed their strength, fostering a growth mindset. I like to take all their pieces and connect them. You can have them share or read the strands anonymously. I like to show them that individually, they have different strengths to bring to the group and that together, we can learn so much from each other. We all have different strengths and that is okay. I even like to share with them things that I am not good at. I tell them that I am not good at soccer, or sports in general. I like to tell them that I cannot draw. They feel empowered that they are better than I am at something. I tell them that throughout the year, I will teach them things that may be a weakness for them. But they can teach me things too and that we will all learn and grow with each other. I mean it, too! Throughout the year, I let them teach *me* at the end of a session or even as the session itself. So much language can be elicited from them teaching others something they are good at.

Famous Failures

Everyone makes mistakes. Even us! I like to tell my students stories about times that I made mistakes, or times when things were challenging for me. How did I feel? What did I do? How did I feel when I overcame those challenges? What did those experiences teach me?

Although students can benefit from hearing our stories, they can also benefit and enjoy learning about celebrities and other famous figures and when they overcame challenges. You can show your students a YouTube video called "Famous Failures," and they can learn about celebrities like Oprah and Michael Jordan. You can have discussions like, would we know about them today if they gave up when things became tough? It is a great way to elicit those conversations and they can see the result of not giving up. Here are some sample discussion questions to use with the video:

- What if Oprah had believed the people who told her she wasn't good enough?
- Can you think of a time you succeeded after failing at first?

Mistake of the Day

One way to normalize making mistakes is by talking about them and realizing that they happen to everyone. You can do this in two ways. You can start each session by having students share a mistake they made in class or outside of the speech room. You can also have students share at the end of a session a mistake they made during the session. You can participate and share your mistakes as well. The benefits are that students will realize that they all have made mistakes and that they are not alone. It is completely normal and even expected that they will get something wrong or do something that they didn't intend to do. But they will also learn the lessons from the mistake. Show them that is even okay to laugh at the mistake. Celebrate mistakes and the lessons learned.

You can also share mistake success stories to normalize the concept further using historical and real-life examples. Include a variety of examples to demonstrate how mistakes have led to groundbreaking achievements. These can inspire students and help normalize mistakes as part of the learning process. Here are some examples you can use.

Successful Failures

Penicillin (Alexander Fleming): Fleming accidentally left out a Petri dish with bacteria, which became contaminated with mold. Instead of discarding it, he noticed the mold killed the bacteria, leading to the discovery of the first antibiotic. **Lesson:** Sometimes, paying attention to accidents can lead to groundbreaking discoveries.

Post-It Notes (Spencer Silver and Art Fry): Spencer Silver accidentally created a weak adhesive while trying to develop a super-strong glue. Years later, Art Fry realized it could be used for bookmarks that wouldn't damage pages, and the Post-It Note was born. **Lesson:** A mistake today might be a solution tomorrow.

Walt Disney: Walt Disney was fired from a newspaper job for "lacking imagination." His first animation studio also went bankrupt. Despite this, he went on to create one of the most successful entertainment companies in the world. **Lesson:** Don't let failure stop you—use it to fuel your next steps.

Thomas Edison: Edison reportedly said, "I have not failed. I've just found 10,000 ways that won't work," when working on the lightbulb. **Lesson:** Perseverance through mistakes can eventually light the way to success.

Michael Jordan: Often cited for saying, "I've missed more than 9,000 shots in my career. I've lost almost 300 games. Twenty-six times I've been trusted to take the game-winning shot and missed. I've failed over and over and over again in my life. And that is why I succeed." **Lesson:** Failure is part of the process to greatness.

J. K. Rowling (*Harry Potter* author): Rowling was rejected by 12 publishers before finally being accepted. Today, her Harry Potter series is one of the best-selling book series of all time. **Lesson:** Sometimes, persistence and believing in your work are the key to success.

Marvel's the Avengers (Robert Downey Jr.): Robert Downey Jr. faced significant personal challenges, including being written off by Hollywood, before turning his life around and becoming Iron Man, a defining role in the Marvel Cinematic Universe. **Lesson:** Mistakes don't define you—how you respond to them does.

Charli D'Amelio (TikTok): Charli has shared stories of failed dance attempts or awkward moments, but she kept practicing and creating. Today, she's one of the most-followed creators on the platform. **Lesson:** Failure is often a natural step to mastering a skill.

Using These Failures

After sharing a story, ask questions to reflect on the lessons:

- What would have happened if Alexander Fleming threw away the contaminated Petri dish?
- How do you think Walt Disney felt after being fired? What might have motivated him to keep going?
- Can you think of a time when something you thought was a failure turned into an opportunity?

By incorporating mistake success stories, paired with activities, reflection prompts, and real-world applications, you can empower students to see mistakes as valuable learning experiences.

Wrong Answers Quiz

You can play a game with your students and encourage them to only provide wrong answers. The game should be low pressure and provide easy questions that they should know the answers to. Model how to give exaggerated and extremely wrong answers, then discuss the correct answers in a positive way. You want to make sure to reward students for participating, not for correct answers.

For example:
Question: What is the fastest land animal?
Funny wrong answer: The tortoise with a jetpack!
Correct answer: The cheetah can run up to 60–70 miles per hour.

Question: What do plants need to grow?
Funny wrong answer: Ice cream and pizza!
Correct answer: Plants need sunlight, water, and air to grow.

Question: How many days are in a week?
Funny wrong answer: A million days!
Correct answer: There are seven days in a week.

These are just a few ways to teach students that making mistakes is normal, expected, and a part of learning. Showing that you make mistakes too will also help with rapport and building trust.

ENCOURAGING A GROWTH MINDSET

This chapter wouldn't be complete without discussing growth mindset. A growth mindset means believing that you can get better at something by trying, learning from mistakes, and practicing. You can explain to your students that it is like thinking of your brain as a muscle that grows stronger when you work hard and don't give up, even when things are tough! You can use analogies like going to the gym and working out to get stronger.

You need to explicitly teach your students the difference between mindsets and why it is important to always strive for a growth mindset. What is the difference between a growth mindset and a fixed mindset? A growth mindset is when you believe you can get better at things by practicing, learning, and not giving up. You know that if something is hard, it just means you need to keep trying. You will improve over time, just like you get better at riding a bike or drawing with practice. A fixed mindset is when you think that you're either good or bad at something, and you can't really change it. People with a fixed mindset might say, "I'm just not good at math," and give up without trying to get better. So, with a growth mindset, you believe you can grow and improve, while with a fixed mindset, you believe your abilities stay the same. It's all about how you think about learning and mistakes! You can use these analogies to demonstrate the difference between the two. Have students discuss times they demonstrated a fixed or growth mindset and the outcomes.

The Power of Yet

One way to encourage having a growth mindset is by teaching the power of yet. Provide your students with conversation scripts and what your inner dialogue should say. Instead of "I can't" they should say "I can't yet." Instead of "I don't know" they should say "I don't know yet." The word "yet" is so powerful. It reminds them that they should not give up and it is not over. Encourage and empower your students to keep trying, even when things get challenging. Practice using this word. You can try role-playing scenarios in which students would have to use "yet" and not give up. You can even show video clips of characters giving up and discuss what would happen if they used "yet" and kept trying. You can even compare two clips, one in which a character gives up and another in which one does not.

The "Yet" Jar

Create a jar where students can add slips of paper with statements they turned from a fixed to a growth mindset using "yet." For example:

- Fixed: "I can't do long division."
- Growth: "I can't do long division yet."

Fixed Mindset Example: Lisa Simpson From *The Simpsons*

Clip: In the episode "Lisa's Sax" (season 9, episode 3), young Lisa initially shows a fixed mindset when she feels defeated by her inability to fit in at school and excel right away in music. She believes that if she can't do something perfectly the first time, she's not talented enough, showing the fixed mindset that talent is static.

Episode: Lisa struggles to overcome her feeling of inadequacy and frustration when she doesn't immediately excel, although she later learns to keep trying.

Growth Mindset Example: *The Flash*

Character: Barry Allen (The Flash)

Clip: In the pilot episode (season 1, episode 1), Barry Allen struggles to control his new powers and fails several times. Despite his early failures, he keeps practicing, learning from each mistake, and improving over time. He admits that he doesn't have it all figured out yet but believes he can improve with effort, showing a growth mindset.

Episode: This is a recurring theme throughout the series, as Barry repeatedly faces challenges but continues to learn, adapt, and grow.

Challenge Chart

Another way to incorporate growth mindset discussions in your speech room is by having a challenge chart. You can create a chart with your students where they list tasks that feel challenging or difficult. These can be tasks such as pronouncing tricky sounds or learning new vocabulary. For each task, students set small goals and track their progress over time. A challenge chart can show students that challenges are opportunities to grow, and that with practice, they can improve. This reinforces the growth mindset idea that effort leads to progress. When introducing it, present hypothetical scenarios and have students brainstorm how to handle them with a growth mindset. For example: "You have a big presentation, but your first attempt didn't go well. What can you do?"

Model and Practice

If you want your students to embody a growth mindset and change the way they respond to challenging tasks, you need to model it and practice it. Give them visuals or sentence strips on what to say instead when things get tough. Such phrases can include "I need help," "I need choices," and "Can I have a hint?" This also shows them that you are there to help them get through the challenging task.

Don't Believe Me?

I asked my SLP Elevate members about their experience with building rapport. One of my members, Elsha Young, provides teletherapy to high school students in Alaska. I asked her about her experience building rapport and making connections with her students. She reported, "So rapport has been absolutely immense. And meeting them where they're at with what they're actually doing, letting them choose their hobbies as therapy themes." Elsha even had a student who never picked up a book show her on a teletherapy session about the anime book he read. He was so excited to have someone to talk about anime with. She also shared, "It's stuff that we all know how to do. If we just give ourselves permission to put down the sticky note, put down the pen and just practice the art of communication at a super basic level. And then you take a progress monitoring, and it's like, boom, we've got it. I've got a couple of kiddos that are AAC users. I've got one that's a seventh grader with eye gaze. She gets on there, and she just giggles and giggles and giggles and giggles. It doesn't matter what I do. And all she does, all we're doing right now is trying to find her spot of where she can actually gaze to activate her device."

NOW WHAT?

I have provided you with several ideas on ways to build rapport and trust with your students. Try one of the suggested activities with your students. They do not require any materials or preparation. Have fun with it, share with your students, laugh with your students, and see how it goes. You may be surprised to find out that you will have fun, too!

Rapport-building dos:

- Be curious about their interests.
- Normalize making mistakes.
- Foster peer connections.

Rapport-building don'ts:

- Don't dismiss their interests, even if they seem trivial to you.
- Avoid judgment when they struggle.

Quick reflection questions:

- What's one thing you could change today to build stronger rapport with your students?
- Do your students feel safe to make mistakes in your speech room? How do you know?

Try this challenge:

- Spend one session focusing solely on rapport-building (no goals or data collection). What do you learn about your students?

8

Routines and Expectations

REWARD SYSTEM GONE WRONG

When I first got a job in a public school, the one thing I was most excited about was having a reward system of my own. After student teaching and working with others' systems, to have my own felt very mature and exciting. At one of my first jobs, when I was working with elementary students, I created gumball machines with construction paper and used fun tack and bingo chips as the gumballs. Remember, this was before Teachers Pay Teachers and fun clip art. I should also inform you that I cannot draw. These were interesting-looking gumballs, but they were mine. Students earned 10 gumballs to get a prize. The gumballs kept falling everywhere, prizes ended up taking so much time to hand out, and I was spending so much money on prizes. But I kept going because I thought that was what I had to do to keep my students participating and behaving.

The following year I got a job with fifth and sixth graders. I had a much larger caseload and did not have enough gumball machines to use. I also didn't think that was appropriate for this age group. I decided to try something different. I decided to have speech dollars and have students earn $10 to get a prize. I found an image of a dollar bill and photocopied a ton of them and spent hours cutting them out. I used library book pockets as the wallets. I let students decorate their wallets the first day of speech and placed all 65 of them on my small therapy wall that I had. I thought this was the best idea in the world. Students wanted to earn money. After a few weeks, I realized this idea was not going to work. Students were complaining that their money in their wallets had gone missing—students were stealing from each other! I was spending my sessions as a detective. I did not have the bandwidth to monitor for thieves and to determine who was being truthful on top of juggling 65 students on my caseload. Looking back, I realize my elaborate reward systems had me focusing more on logistics than on my students' actual progress. Sure, rewards can work for some students, but they're not a magic fix for participation or engagement. That's when I started to realize the importance of routines and expectations as a foundation for success.

To Reward or Not to Reward

After my reward system failed me, I realized I had to find another system or throw it out altogether. Did my students really need rewards to get them to participate? This made me think about intrinsic and extrinsic motivation. Using rewards was working somewhat to get my students extrinsically motivated. But was it working for all my students? No. Some of them did not care at all about the dollars and prizes. Some just wanted the prizes, didn't even participate, and would get mad or combative if their peers all got a prize and they did not. I was also spending a ton of money and time on prizes, and I only had students for 30 minutes once or twice a week.

I needed to find a way to get them intrinsically motivated. How could I show them that learning can be fun? How could I show them that they could be successful with me? How could I show them that what we were doing was relevant to their world? Classroom teachers can use grades on a report card as a motivator. SLPs don't have that luxury. We need a different approach. We need to explicitly teach students and not be afraid to talk about it often. That is where routines and expectations come in.

WHAT DO YOU EXPECT?

Before I can discuss how to teach your students about expectations in your speech room, you need to decide what you expect of them. Expectations are like the foundation of a house. Without them, everything you try to build—whether it's trust, progress, or even just participation—becomes shaky and unstable. A solid foundation of clear rules and expectations ensures that your speech room can withstand challenges, whether it's a tough day for a student or an unexpected disruption. Brainstorm some expectations for speech. There are no wrong answers. How do you feel about the following:

- Are they coming on their own or are you coming to get them?
- What happens if they forget to come to speech?

- What do they need to bring with them?
- Should they wait outside the room once they get there or come in quietly?
- What should they do once they enter the room?
- Where should they sit?
- What should they do when others are taking a turn or answering a question?
- Do they need to raise their hand or just wait to be called upon?
- What should they do if they make a mistake?
- What happens at the end of the session? Do they wait to be dismissed? Wait for the bell?

By thinking about these answers, you can consider what works best for you, your students, and the building you work in. Everyone's situations will be different, but what is most important is for you to determine what works best for you. What expectations have worked well for you in the past? What challenges have you faced in setting or enforcing them?

Here are some of the expectations that I set for my fifth and sixth graders:

- All students, other than my life skill students, can come to speech on their own, unless they have lost their privileges.
- If they forget to come to speech, depending on the location of their classrooms and other logistics, I use the intercom to remind them to attend, or go and pick them up.
- They only need to bring their Chromebooks to speech unless they have lost that privilege.
- I keep all writing utensils and supplies in the speech room for them.
- I keep a folder in the speech room for them to hold any work that we do. The folder stays in my office so that I can refer to it to remind myself what we accomplished. I also do not want them forgetting it or losing it in their classrooms.
- If I put a sign on my door that says "speech cancelled" they should return to class because I am stuck in a meeting.
- If my door is closed and I am still working with other students, they should wait quietly in the hallway.
- They should enter the speech room quietly and take a seat, any seat, since there are no assigned seats. (Even though they may insist that they sit in the same seat every session. I even made sure I found five of the same exact chairs so that no one felt they had a better chair.)
- Everyone will get a turn, let everyone speak, and don't make fun if others need more help or make a mistake.

- During games, everyone will get a turn. It isn't based on getting an answer right or wrong, because everyone will get it right.
- At the end of a session, put any work in the folders, put away any pencils, and wait to be dismissed.

Those were my expectations of my students in my speech room. It was what worked for me after trying many different things over the years. Your expectations may change too and that is okay! Here are some other things to consider:

- **Arrive on time:** Be seated and ready to begin when class starts.
- **Respect the space:** Keep the room tidy and treat materials and equipment with care.
- **Be respectful:** Listen attentively when others are speaking or performing.
- **Follow instructions:** Pay attention to the teacher's directions and any posted rules.
- **Bring necessary materials:** Always have your speech, notes, and any required props.
- **Participate actively:** Engage in all activities, whether performing or offering feedback.
- **Use appropriate language:** Speak professionally and kindly during all discussions.
- **Practice professionalism:** Maintain good posture, eye contact, and clear speech when speaking.
- **Collaborate:** Work well with peers during group activities or critiques.
- **Stay positive:** Offer constructive feedback and support your classmates' efforts.

Remember, it doesn't matter what you decide. Just be mindful of your students' ages and make expectations and rules appropriate for them.

YOU HAVE RULES AND EXPECTATIONS. . .NOW WHAT?

You have decided on the expectations for your students. You now need to build routines so that students know what is expected of them on a regular basis. You need to explicitly teach them and remind them of what they should and should not do in the speech room. You cannot expect to tell them once, put a poster on the wall, and expect them to remember and follow through. It may take you a few sessions of reviewing it.

For example, for my first session with my speech students, I would pick them up from their classrooms. I did not expect them to know when their session was yet or where to go. I would remind them how to walk in the hallways together. When we got to my speech room, I would show them how to wait in the hallway if needed, how to enter the room appropriately, and even show them my "speech cancelled" sign and discussed what to do if they saw that on my door. Then, we practiced entering my speech room and finding a seat. We would decorate their speech folders and show them where they would find them in the speech room. We would discuss what to do when the session ends and even practice it if necessary. For some students or groups, I might have to remind them of all these things the first few sessions. It is worth the time to put in the beginning to set the stage for the rest of the school year.

Here are some quick low-prep strategies for teaching routines:

- **Role-playing:** Practice entering and leaving the room, asking for help, or responding to feedback.
- **Visual supports:** Create posters or cards with key routines.
- **Cueing:** Use hand signals or prompts to remind students of rules in the moment.
- **Gamify it:** Turn routine practice into a game—for example, awarding points to the group for following rules.

Creating routines in your speech room will help in so many ways. Students will know what is expected of them, they will feel less overwhelmed, and there will be more time to work on goals and have fun. Think of routines as a GPS for your speech room. Without them, students wander aimlessly, unsure of where they're going or how to get there. With clear routines in place, they know exactly what steps to take and feel confident navigating even unfamiliar tasks. Just like a GPS reduces travel stress, routines reduce anxiety and confusion, helping students focus on the journey of learning.

The Benefits of Rules and Expectations

Creating rules, expectations, and routines provides several important benefits when it comes to working with secondary speech students. Younger speech students can benefit from these too. This section discusses how rules and routines benefit older students. Creating rules and expectations:

Establishes a Positive Learning Environment

Clear rules and expectations set the tone for respect and collaboration. When students understand what is expected, they feel safer and more comfortable participating. This can reduce anxiety, especially in speech when students can be embarrassed to be there and very aware of their learning and communication difficulties. I had a student who was extremely shy and barely spoke during our first few sessions. By setting the expectation that everyone in the group got a turn and that mistakes were okay, he slowly started participating. One day, he surprised the entire group by confidently answering a question without hesitation. When I asked him later what helped, he said, "I just knew no one here would laugh at me." That's when I knew the power of clear, supportive expectations.

Promotes Consistency and Structure

Routines give students a predictable framework. Predictability can reduce uncertainty and help students focus on the task at hand. Knowing what comes next helps secondary students stay on track and minimizes off-task behavior. My Monday morning group used to feel like herding cats—students wandered in late, sat wherever they wanted, and interrupted constantly. After introducing a clear routine—enter quietly, grab your folder, and sit at the therapy table—everything changed. Now, they arrive ready to start, and we can get through a full lesson without losing half the session to chaos.

Encourages Responsibility and Accountability

When rules and expectations are clear, students learn to take responsibility for their own behavior. They understand the consequences of their actions. This can help them develop self-discipline, which can impact them outside of the speech room as well. One year, I worked with a student who frequently forgot to bring her Chromebook to speech. Instead of getting frustrated, I added a routine where every student got a reminder pass for their sessions and what to bring. After a few weeks, this student started showing up prepared every time. She even helped remind another student in the group who almost forgot something.

Fosters Respectful Communication

A structured environment promotes active listening, respectful feedback, and effective communication. These are critical skills not only for speech but for students' overall academic and personal development. During a group session, one of my students would always cut off another student when she was answering. After introducing a hand-raising system and setting the rule that everyone deserves a chance to speak, the dynamic shifted. This student began participating more, and the other student learned to wait his turn.

Reduces Behavioral Issues

With clear expectations, students know the boundaries of acceptable behavior, which can decrease disruptions. A well-managed speech therapy room allows for more time on task, which is especially important in a subject where participation and practice are essential. I had a student who often interrupted others during group discussions. After introducing clear expectations about turn-taking and practicing them as a group, he started to wait his turn more consistently—because he understood the routine and felt confident in his role.

Boosts Confidence

When students know the rules and routines, they can better prepare and anticipate their role in our therapy rooms. This predictability boosts their confidence, making them more willing to perform in front of their peers and take risks in their learning. I'll never forget one of my students, who always panicked when I asked him to answer questions in front of the group. After introducing a rule that allowed students to pass and come back to a question, he started participating more. Eventually, he stopped passing altogether and even volunteered to answer first sometimes. He told me later, "I just needed time to think first, and knowing I could pass made it less scary."

Promotes Active Participation

When students understand the routines, they are more likely to participate actively. As students know when and how to contribute effectively, they will be more willing to participate in discussions and respond to feedback. Once my students knew the routine—that everyone gets a turn, and mistakes are okay—they started engaging more freely. The predictability helped them relax and focus on the task instead of worrying about "messing up."

Reduces Anxiety

Routines provide predictability, which is especially important for secondary students who may feel nervous about getting things wrong in front of their peers. When students know what to expect, they can focus more on their performance and less on the uncertainty of what's coming next. One of my students had severe anxiety and would freeze if she thought she'd get something wrong in front of the group. By setting a routine where everyone answered questions at their own pace, and mistakes were normalized as part of learning, she started engaging more. One day, she told me, "I like coming here because I don't feel like I have to be perfect." That simple reassurance made all the difference.

Enhances Time Management

Consistent routines allow for efficient use of therapy time. This helps maximize learning opportunities and keeps the session moving at a steady pace. We only have students for a limited time. We want to make sure we are using time wisely. I had a Friday group that always seemed to start late because students would drift in one by one, chatting about their weekend plans. After setting the rule that sessions started promptly at the bell and introducing a quick warm-up activity, we gained back 10 minutes of teaching time every week. That extra time made a huge difference in helping the group hit their goals by the end of the year.

You want your students to participate. You want them to feel safe. You want them to be willing to take risks in front of their peers. Your students are aware of their difficulties. By implementing and adhering to rules, expectations, and routines, the secondary speech room can become a space where students can thrive both academically and personally. How do you currently teach routines in your speech room? What's one new idea you'd like to try?

LET'S GIVE THEM A SAY

This chapter would not be complete if I did not take the time to discuss the benefits of giving your students a say. You can give them a say in various aspects of your sessions: how they arrive, materials they use, and ways they are reinforced. When you give them a say, you are empowering them and fostering ownership of their learning. You want them to have intrinsic motivation. You want them to want to be there and not just be there and participate because you said so. This is another way you can make this happen. Giving students a say in the rules and routines is like coauthoring a contract. When they're part of the process, they're more likely to honor the agreement because they've helped write it. It's no longer just "your" speech room—it becomes a shared space where everyone has ownership and accountability.

When I started with older students, I was young and naïve. I wanted my students to respect me because that was what I thought we had to do. I was a teacher in a building that was demanding respect, and I felt like I had to play along. I told them to come to speech, I told them where to sit, I told them to participate, and I even told them to have fun. It was all about what I wanted. I could not understand why they weren't motivated and didn't want to do what I said.

As part of my journey to learning how to better serve my older students, learn what they needed, and learn how to motivate them, I also reflected on motivation. Giving them a say in various aspects is an easy way to get their buy-in and willingness to work with us, not for us.

Here are some examples of ways to give students a say:

- **Choice of writing utensils:** Let students decide if they want to use pencils, colored pens, markers, or even dry-erase boards when working on any written expression activity. I like to have a drawer filled with options. My students' fan favorite was scented gel pens.
- **Choose how they are reminded about speech:** Allow students to choose how they prefer to be reminded about their speech sessions—whether it's through a written note, an email, a class announcement, or a calendar app reminder.
- **Topic or theme selection:** Give students options to pick topics or themes they are interested in and use them for articulation or language goals. This makes the session more engaging and relevant to their interests.
- **Choice of reinforcement:** Let students have a say in how they are rewarded for their effort—whether it's verbal praise, stickers, extra free time, or another form of positive reinforcement. This doesn't mean you have to have a reward system or prize bin. But knowing how they like to be rewarded can be used when needed. My students often liked to just have time to listen to music at the end of the session or free time on their Chromebooks.
- **Flexible seating options:** Allow students to choose where they sit during sessions—whether it's a traditional desk, a bean bag chair, or standing at a podium, giving them a level of comfort while they practice. I understand that not all speech rooms have the space to incorporate true flexible seating. My room did not. I would let my students stand if they needed to and not criticize them if they needed to sit on their feet.
- **Choose how feedback is delivered:** Let students choose whether they prefer to receive feedback. You cannot assume that every student will be comfortable getting feedback in front of their peers. Maybe consider a hand signal that reminds a student to repeat their articulation target. Maybe a short one-on-one discussion at the end of a session. Find out what your students prefer.
- **To read or not to read:** Do they have read out loud in your speech room? I always like to remind my students that I am not there to embarrass them. When we are doing a reading activity, I always ask if they want to read without pressure. They always know and can trust that I will read it to them if they would prefer.

■ **Give speech therapy a new name:** Do they want to refer to your room as "speech?" They may find that it sounds immature or doesn't accurately reflect what they are working on with you. Maybe give them the option to call your class something different. Some suggestions could be Language Lab, Communication Zone, or even just your name or room number.

These are just some ideas and suggestions that you can use to give your students more of a say during their speech therapy sessions. By giving students a voice in their speech therapy sessions, you can create a more personalized, motivating, and engaging learning environment. If you are rigid with them, they will be less willing to work hard and take risks when tasks become challenging.

Remember, you can't always know what happens before a session or during the day. You can only control what goes on in your speech room. The more you can make your students feel comfortable, the more they will be willing to share with you and participate despite other challenges they are having. Although you should have routines, you should also be flexible and adapt when necessary. If you are too rigid, you will miss opportunities for your students to trust you and feel comfortable.

YOUR ACTION PLAN

1. Identify your top three expectations.
2. Draft a simple, age-appropriate way to introduce them to students.
3. Pick one way to involve students in creating or practicing routines.
4. Implement and refine as needed—be flexible and patient.

NOW WHAT?

Now that I have discussed how to create rules, expectations, and routines, it is time for you to brainstorm and implement. You don't need a Pinterest-perfect set of rules and routines—just something that works and doesn't have you chasing imaginary speech dollars all day. What are some things you are already doing that can be made more official as a rule? Are you discussing this often and on a regular basis? What are ways you can give your students a say in their speech sessions? Can you incorporate new or more ways to give them a say on a regular basis? Take the time to practice and review these things often. I promise, it won't take time away from working on goals and collecting data. Remember, if you want data to collect, you need your students to know what to expect.

3

The 60-Minute Plan Strategy

In this section, which includes Chapters 9 through 14, I share practical tips and tricks so that you can plan for your entire caseload (no matter what the size) in an hour a week. Yes, it is possible to plan that quickly and still be effective. I also discuss how to prepare and execute a lesson for mixed groups. When you can plan quickly and easily, you have so much more time for yourself and for other aspects of the job. Dive in to see how!

A Plan for Work-Life Balance

Picture this: it's 9:00 pm, and I'm sitting at my kitchen table, surrounded by a sea of laminating sheets, colored markers, and half-finished reports. My dinner is cold, my to-do list is endless, and I'm asking myself, "Is this what being an SLP is supposed to feel like?" Spoiler alert: It's not. But early in my career, I thought it was the only way to succeed. I thought every lesson, every goal, needed a unique plan and new resources to target it. It was all I knew how to do, and I thought that was the only way to get the job done. I was not taught anything different in graduate school. I was a new SLP and luckily did not have many demands outside of work, which allowed me to have that time. That said, I knew it would not be sustainable in the long run.

As years went on, my caseload became larger, and with that came new challenges of even more paperwork, more demands, and less time. To add to the mix, I had new challenges outside of work. My husband and I were ready to start a family and that lead to fertility issues. I found myself driving to my doctor in the morning before work. I knew stress management was essential and important in order to be successful with that journey. Luckily, we were successful, but then I had to juggle being a working mother and could not take work home like I was able to in the past.

Work-life balance isn't about juggling perfectly—it's about knowing which balls can bounce and which ones will break if you drop them. When I started, I treated every task like it was made of glass—spending hours laminating, lesson planning, and perfecting every detail. Over time, I realized it's okay to let some things go, if I'm focusing on what truly matters. I learned many lessons in these phases of my life about work-life balance and how to manage my time so that I could leave work at work and not let work take over my life. I used these lessons to help those graduate clinicians I worked with to teach them about time management to help set them up for success later in their careers. I hope to help others learn from mistakes I have made so that they can feel less stressed and enjoy the work they are doing more.

TIME IS MONEY

When I was in my undergraduate program, I had a professor that taught diagnostics by always saying, "time is money." I didn't know why, but that line stuck with me so much. Maybe because she scared me into never coming late to class even though it was 8 am (and we know that is not easy for a college kid). But once I entered the field, I still remembered what that professor used to drill into us. I did not embody that belief. I clearly didn't understand what my professor meant. I worked through lunch, stayed late after school, and brought home endless piles of paperwork—only to feel constantly behind. It wasn't until I realized I was spending more time managing *tasks* than enjoying my work or my life that it clicked. Time really is money—because it's a currency you can never get back. As I became a seasoned clinician, I realized how valuable time is. There are only so many hours in a day. If you want to leave work at work and not bring a ton home, you need to prioritize and use your time wisely.

Time is money, as they say—and let me tell you, I spent way too much time being broke in my early career. My first year as an SLP was basically me throwing wads of time into the laminator and hoping something stuck. Spoiler alert: It didn't.

You aren't getting paid overtime to bring work home or work through your lunch periods. You need to make sure you are maximizing your time. You can think differently about your planning and paperwork to ensure you save time and energy. If you get burned out, you won't be fully present to serve your students. You won't be present outside of work either. Work might be a big part of your life, but it shouldn't be your entire life. Only you can put yourself first.

PRIORITIZING: MANAGING THE CHAOS

Deciding what to prioritize can be tricky, when there are so many tasks, so many things, and they all seem so important. Think about what you need to do right now and what you can leave for the next day. Do you need to plan individual activities for every lesson, or can you take one activity and use it with as many groups as possible?

When you're an SLP, everything feels urgent. There's the report that's due tomorrow, the parent email you haven't answered yet, the therapy session you still need to plan, and the stack of paperwork piling up on your desk. With so much demanding your attention, how do you decide what needs to get done first?

Using the Eisenhower Matrix

Enter the *Eisenhower Matrix*—a simple but powerful tool to help you manage your time effectively by categorizing tasks based on urgency and importance. The Eisenhower Matrix, named after former U.S. President Dwight D. Eisenhower, divides tasks into four quadrants based on two key criteria: urgency and importance. Here's how it works:

Quadrant 1: Urgent and Important (Do it now)

These are the tasks that demand your immediate attention and have serious consequences if left undone. For example:

- Writing a report for tomorrow's IEP meeting.
- Completing Medicaid billing before the monthly deadline.

> **TIP**
>
> Tackle these tasks first thing in your day when your energy is highest.

Quadrant 2: Important but Not Urgent (Plan it)

These tasks contribute to your long-term success but don't need immediate attention. For example:

- Preparing for an evaluation that's due in two weeks.
- Creating templates to streamline your report writing.

> **TIP**
>
> Schedule time in your calendar for these tasks before they become urgent.

Quadrant 3: Urgent but Not Important (Delegate it)

These tasks may feel pressing but don't require your unique skills. For example:

- A colleague asking for a quick favor that takes you off-task.
- Handling routine scheduling requests that an assistant or software could manage.

> **TIP**
>
> If possible, delegate or find systems to handle these tasks.

Quadrant 4: Not Urgent and Not Important (Eliminate it)

These are the distractions that add no value to your goals. For example:

- Spending hours scrolling Pinterest for therapy ideas you don't need right now.
- Perfecting the formatting of a report that's already functional.

> **TIP**
>
> Let these tasks go. They're not worth your time.

Using the Eisenhower Matrix doesn't mean you need to spend hours categorizing every task. It's about developing a mindset to quickly assess what matters most. Here's how I use it:

1. **Make a daily task list:** Start your day by writing down everything you need to accomplish.
2. **Sort tasks into quadrants:** Ask yourself two questions:
   - Is this urgent?
   - Is this important?
   Then place each task in the appropriate quadrant.
3. **Focus on Quadrant 1 first:** Tackle urgent and important tasks before anything else.
4. **Block time for Quadrant 2:** Schedule time for tasks that are important but not urgent. This is where you grow professionally and stay ahead of deadlines.
5. **Pass off Quadrant 3:** These tasks feel urgent, but they're not truly important. Don't let them hijack your day. When possible, delegate, defer, or create a system to handle them without your constant involvement. Protect your time for what really moves the needle.
6. **Say no to Quadrant 4:** Recognize what can be eliminated entirely and don't be afraid to let it go.

Let me share how the Eisenhower Matrix saved me during a particularly hectic week:

- **Quadrant 1:** A progress report due by end-of-day for a high-stakes IEP meeting. This went straight to the top of my list, and I dedicated my morning to finishing it.
- **Quadrant 2:** Preparing visuals for a big group therapy session happening next week. It wasn't urgent, but I blocked time on my calendar to work on it later in the week.
- **Quadrant 3:** Answering a last-minute question from a teacher about scheduling. I quickly forwarded it to the administrative assistant to handle.
- **Quadrant 4:** Rewriting a lesson plan that was already good enough. I reminded myself that "perfect" wasn't necessary, and I moved on.

By the end of the day, I felt accomplished and far less overwhelmed, knowing I'd tackled what mattered most.

The beauty of the Eisenhower Matrix is that it can be adapted to fit your workflow. It's not about perfection; it's about clarity. When you know what to prioritize, you free up mental energy to focus on what truly matters, not just at work but in your personal life, too.

Take a moment to reflect: What's one task on your plate today that belongs in Quadrant 2? How can you schedule it to avoid the last-minute scramble? By using the Eisenhower Matrix, you'll find yourself making progress with less stress—and more time for you.

The 60-Minute Plan Strategy

This section discusses how to plan in one hour a week or less. Yes, it is possible. It won't make you a bad clinician or appear lazy. It will allow you to work smarter not harder and have more time for yourself outside of work. This will help with work-life balance and prevent burn out. At first, the idea of planning in an hour felt impossible. But when I started using one activity across multiple groups, it was a game-changer. One week, I used a single set of task cards to target main ideas, summarizing, and inferencing for three different groups. I adjusted the questions slightly for each group and was done. An hour of planning turned into a full week of lessons.

This strategy is all about looking at materials and activities differently. How many goals can you address with these materials and activities? How can you change your questioning or approach to meet a variety of needs? Think of planning as a puzzle. Each piece—an activity, a strategy, or a material—can fit multiple goals and needs if you look at it creatively. For example, one set of task cards can address main ideas for one group, summarizing for another, and inferencing for yet another. You don't need a new piece for every goal; just find different ways to use the pieces you already have. Be adaptable and flexible and think outside of the box.

By planning quickly, easily, and confidently, you can devote more of the little precious time you have for report writing and other paperwork aspects of the job that we cannot avoid. Here are some tips for saving time with paperwork:

- Use templates to save time with evaluation reports. I am not saying write the same thing for everyone, but how can you use frequent report descriptions or even common results explanations and make templates for yourself?
- How can you plan and be prepared? You know the due dates ahead of time for annual reviews and tentative meeting dates. I like to do this at the beginning of the year when I receive a caseload. Mark down dates on a calendar. But also mark down when you need to test for reevaluations, when you need to start writing reports, when you need to work on IEPs. Mark it all down and hold yourself accountable. Don't just mark down due dates but mark down dates to get things done. Leave yourself wiggle room since we all know things come up, like kids absent on the day you planned to test them. I know I don't do well with last-minute tasks, so I like to map things out so that I have time and wiggle room.
- Make all necessary photocopies and documents ahead of time. Do you send home surveys or checklists before meetings? Have those ready and photocopied or even labeled and ready to go at the beginning of the year so that you are pre-pared when things get busy and hectic.

These are just some ways you can cut down time and feel prepared with the paperwork aspects of the job. The more you can do when things are calm at the beginning of the year, the better. Your future self will thank you.

STAY INSPIRED, NOT TIRED

By planning quickly and easily, you can avoid the dreaded burnout. By keeping energy high, you can stay inspired. If you struggle with this, always remember your why. Why did you become an SLP? Why did you decide to work in the schools? Why did you work with this age group? What impact are you having on your students?

If you are having trouble answering some of these questions, I recommend reflecting if you are having enough time to be inspired. Are you celebrating your wins? You are an amazing SLP (or future SLP) just by reading this book, and your students (or future students) are so lucky to have you. Celebrate that. Remember that.

Self-care is essential. You can't keep running on empty and expect to be your very best. Whether it's taking a walk, reading a book, or just zoning out with Netflix, those moments of rest aren't indulgent—they're necessary to keep you going. You cannot pour from an empty cup, so you want to make sure you take care of yourself and have time for you outside of work.

Make sure you build routines for yourself to incorporate fun hobbies, exercise, or whatever else is important to you. Even if you are early on in your career and do not have kids at home to worry about, still work on trying to reduce the need to bring work home so that you have things in place for when life outside of work changes. Yes, it may take time to build some things in the beginning. It is very common to take more work home in the early years or have things take more time like report writing. The more you do it the easier it will become. You will get stronger. You will know how to find things faster and how to use things in a variety of ways, so you don't need a million materials to be successful.

MISTAKES SLPs MAKE

I have made many of these mistakes myself over the years and have seen many others make similar mistakes. You can learn from my mistakes and get to the other side faster. Maybe you have found yourself making one or all of these mistakes. That is okay. That doesn't make you a bad SLP. But if work-life balance is important for you, I recommend considering some of the following ways to avoid these mistakes:

Overthinking

Raise your hand if you've ever spent an hour Googling "creative therapy ideas," opened 27 tabs, pinned 15 activities to Pinterest, and then realized it was bedtime, and you hadn't planned a thing. If that's you, welcome to the club—I'm the president. SLPs are perfectionists. We don't like to be wrong. We have our students' and clients' best interest at heart. We want to know we are making a difference and helping them. We spend so much time wondering what to do with them that we take longer to plan and prepare. We get into our heads. You second guess yourself and spend too much time and energy planning and still feel unsure of yourself. Instead, I recommend going with your gut. Activities don't need to be fancy or elaborate to be effective. Just take something, anything, and go with it. What is the worst that can happen? It doesn't go as planned. Learn from it and move on. Your students also won't know or care if it didn't go as planned.

Overplanning

Early on, I planned every session like it was a Broadway show—props, scripts, costumes (okay, maybe not costumes). Now I know my students don't need a production; they need consistency and clarity. Can you relate? You plan too many activities for one session. You plan a different activity for each group or session. This leaves you with so many activities. Remember, more stuff does not mean more or better results. Instead, how can you use one activity with as many groups or goals as possible? How can you use one activity or resource other than how it was intended? Your students won't care that you used a main idea activity to also work on summarizing. Planning a session is like following a recipe—less is more. You don't need 20 ingredients (or activities) to make a great dish. Stick to a few key components, and you'll create something just as effective without the stress of juggling too many tasks.

Being Disorganized

You forget what resources you have planned. You forget what resources you already have. You are feeling frazzled and unprepared. Fewer materials will help you feel less disorganized and less frazzled. This is coming from a type B SLP.

SETTING BOUNDARIES: THE KEY TO SUSTAINABLE SUCCESS

Setting boundaries is one of the most important (and overlooked) components of maintaining work-life balance as an SLP. It's not just about protecting your personal time—it's about preserving your energy and ensuring you show up as your best self for both your students and yourself.

Think of boundaries as the walls around you to protect you. They protect your time and energy from being overtaken by unnecessary demands, allowing you to focus on what truly matters. Without boundaries, it's easy to feel pulled in every direction, constantly saying "yes" to things that drain you and leave little time for yourself.

Boundaries are so important. With increasing caseloads, school districts struggling to find SLPs, and budget cuts, you can only do so much. Boundaries matter because they:

- **Protect your time and energy:** Saying "no" to tasks that don't align with your priorities gives you more bandwidth for the things that truly matter—whether that's delivering high-quality therapy or spending time with your family.

- **Prevent burnout:** Constantly overextending yourself can lead to exhaustion and resentment, making it harder to stay passionate about your work.
- **Model healthy habits:** When you set boundaries, you teach your colleagues, students, and even yourself that it's okay to prioritize well-being.

The following section lists some practical ways you can set boundaries for yourself. I cannot say I have been successful with all of these, but I can at least say I tried. Refer to this section if you are ever in any of these situations.

Establish Work Hours and Stick to Them

Decide when your workday ends and resist the urge to check emails or tackle paperwork outside those hours. If something comes up after hours, it can likely wait until the next day.

Example: "I leave work at 4:30 pm every day. My email notifications are off after that, so I'm not tempted to reply to messages from home."

Say No (Gracefully)

You don't have to accept every request that comes your way. If something doesn't align with your role or priorities, politely decline or delegate.

Example: "I'd love to help, but my schedule is packed this week. Is there someone else who could assist?"

Create a Physical Workspace

If you're working from home or catching up on paperwork, designate a specific area for work. When you leave that space, leave the work behind.

Example: "I work at the kitchen table, but I clear everything away when I'm done, so it doesn't linger in my mind—or my space."

Limit Your Availability

If you're always available, people will assume they can interrupt you anytime. Set clear boundaries for when and how you can be contacted.

Example: "I check my emails twice a day: once in the morning and once after lunch. If it's urgent, please call me directly."

Build in Buffer Time

Schedule breaks between sessions or meetings to reset and recharge. This prevents you from feeling rushed or overwhelmed. This is also when I run to the bathroom without feeling like I am taking time away from students' sessions.

Example: "I schedule 10-minute 'transition times' between sessions to gather my materials and take a breather."

If setting boundaries feels selfish, remind yourself that it's the opposite. Boundaries help you preserve your energy so you can give your best to the things—and people—that matter most. Think of it this way: you wouldn't run a marathon without pacing yourself, so why should your workday be any different?

Communicating Your Needs

As SLPs that are experts in communication, we can find it a challenge to communicate our own wants and needs. We are natural people pleasers. I encourage you to be proactive and clear when sharing your boundaries with others.

- With colleagues: "I'm happy to collaborate, but I need a few days' notice to fit it into my schedule."
- With administrators: "I'm available for after-school meetings on Wednesdays, but I keep my other evenings open for family commitments."
- With yourself: "I won't stay at work past 5:00 pm, even if my to-do list isn't finished. There's always tomorrow."

MY LESSON PLANNING TIPS

One question I get asked often is what is necessary to jot down in a planner or to feel prepared for a session. You don't have to write elaborate lesson plans for every session. SLP sessions are unique, to meet the unique needs of our students. Often administrators ask us to submit lesson plans ahead of time. The problem with this is that we don't know how our students will do. Therefore, we don't know what we will need to do in the next session based on how they did.

Here are things that I like to jot down to plan for a session. As years have gone on, I don't need to be as thorough with my plans. I can just jot down one or two words in a planner to help me recall my game plan. You can get access to a sample plan format sheet on my free supplemental resources page for this book at www.speechtimefun.com/book.

- **Goal:** The annual goal(s) being addressed in the session.
- **Session objective:** The benchmark or mini goal am I addressing. Remember, you don't want to be addressing that annual goal each session throughout the year. There are tasks needed to eventually be successful with that annual goal.
- **Introduction:** How am I introducing the lesson? How am I showing my students the WHY we are doing what we are doing? How is this relevant to them?
- **Strategy:** How am I teaching the skill? How am I teaching my students explicitly how to be successful with the task at hand? How am I using their strengths to compensate for their weaknesses? We covered these various strategies in Section 1 of this book.
- **Activity/materials:** What do I need to be prepared? What is the ONE activity that the entire session will be based around? I may need different follow-up activities or visual aids for the different needs of the group.
- **Conclusion:** How am I wrapping up the session? How am I reminding them of what they learned, how they can use it outside of the speech room, and how is this relevant to them? This is the opportunity to remind students of the wins they had during the session.

These additional practical tips can help simplify your lesson planning and make the process even smoother. These strategies will help you feel prepared without overcomplicating things, giving you more time to focus on what truly matters:

- **Take advantage of digital tools:** Use technology to save time and stay organized.
  - Example: Apps like Google Slides can create interactive lessons, while tools like Google Keep or OneNote can store and organize your planning notes and ideas.
  - Pro tip: Save templates for digital resources you can tweak each session instead of starting from scratch.
- **Batch-plan for efficiency:** Set aside time weekly or monthly to batch-plan multiple sessions. This is more efficient than planning day by day.
  - Example: Spend one hour on Friday planning all of next week's sessions.
  - Pro tip: Keep it simple—choose a core activity or resource and plan variations for different groups.
- **Keep a "Plan B" kit:** Life happens—students are absent, or a lesson takes less time than expected. Have a stash of easy-to-implement backup activities ready to go.
  - Example: Printable word puzzles, card games, or a quick YouTube video discussion.
  - Pro tip: Include materials that can target a variety of goals, so they're versatile.

- **Keep it simple:** Remember, planning doesn't need to be elaborate to be effective. Sometimes, a single worksheet, a discussion, or a set of task cards is all you need.
  - Example: Take an article from Readworks.org and use it to target a variety of goals. Just click Print! Create a cheat sheet of questions to ask that you can refer to. This doesn't need to be a cute cheat sheet, just a piece of paper!
  - Pro tip: Focus on quality over quantity—students will benefit more from well-executed simplicity than from an overly complex plan.

NOW WHAT?

It is reflection time! Take some time to reflect and think about these questions and prompts. Reflect on your time management and prioritizing skills. Reflect on your work-life balance.

- How would you currently rate your work-life balance, from 1 (needs major improvement) to 5 (you have it all figured out)?
- Take 10 minutes to write down three things that stress you out most about your current workload. Then, brainstorm one small change you can make to address each one.
- Make a goal for yourself. What is one aspect you can work on first to make improvements in your rating score?
- If you had more time for yourself, what would you do with that time? Remember, it doesn't make you a bad SLP. We are all a work in progress.

I hope after taking time to think and reflect, you realize that we have all made mistakes and have room to grow. Self-care and prioritizing time management are essential to getting the job done and continuing to love what you do each day. You are making such an impact, and your students are so lucky to have you. They need you to show up for them each day. They need you. Remember, work-life balance isn't a luxury—it's a necessity. You deserve to feel fulfilled in your work and your personal life. Start small, be consistent, and give yourself grace along the way.

10

Feeling Relevant Without Using the Curriculum

If you've ever felt like a glorified tutor, you're not alone. Early in my career, I thought relevance in speech therapy meant staying glued to the classroom curriculum. It took a lot of frustration—and reflection—for me to realize that we have the flexibility and creativity to approach relevance in a way that truly helps our students thrive. I always thought that to have relevant lessons, I had to incorporate the curriculum. I remember working at a high school for the first time. I did not understand why these students were receiving speech and language services. I did not know why they had been given some of their goals. I remember working individually with a tenth grader. It was an individual session only because no other students were available at that time. She was quiet and reserved. She did not ask for help or even engage in much conversation with me. She had vocabulary goals, so I decided to just take her science vocabulary and add visual aids and simplified definitions. She did not complain, and that was all I really did. I did not feel like I made a massive impact or was setting her up for success. Yes, she was feeling more confident with science, but what about the other subjects? I did not even teach her how to do this for herself so she could be successful without me. I was just trying to fill the time and get the job done.

Maybe you can relate to this experience. We want to make a difference and impact and know that our sessions are valuable. I had to reflect on this experience. The more I thought about this, the more I realized that our students need strategies to help them access the curriculum. I decided to try other approaches. I tried using materials that were at their level. I started writing my own passages and questions. I used simplified language. I used their interests. I started seeing more engagement, more progress, and we had more fun. I realized I didn't need to use curriculum to get results, I just had to have the right materials and the right approach.

Learning is hard for these students, and we can be relevant in so many other ways. Feeling like a glorified tutor? It's time to rethink what relevance means in speech therapy. You don't need to be an expert in every subject or a walking textbook. Your superpower is teaching the skills that empower students to succeed across all subjects.

THE BENEFITS OF BREAKING FREE FROM CURRICULUM

To have the biggest impact, you need to follow a plan and be strategic. You want your lessons to yield results, so you need a plan. You want your lessons to be relevant, but you don't need to stick with the curriculum to do so.

By focusing lessons on the language and communication skills students need, you can help them access the curriculum and participate in classroom activities. Curriculum objectives are typically extremely language heavy, with challenging vocabulary, usually above students' reading levels—and boring. If you bring these objectives into your speech sessions, you are setting your students up for failure and for avoidance. Research shows that students often struggle with classroom content because of underlying language weaknesses—not the content itself. Strengthening those foundational skills can have a bigger impact than just tutoring them through the material.

Working on language skills helps students access the classroom curriculum in the following ways:

- **Enhances reading comprehension:** Language skills are foundational for understanding written texts. Improving vocabulary, syntax, and inferencing abilities helps students comprehend complex passages, follow plot developments, and understand informational texts. These skills are crucial for success in subjects like English, social studies, and science.
- **Improves ability to follow directions:** Strong receptive language skills enable students to understand and follow multistep directions, which is essential for participating in class activities, completing assignments, and following procedural tasks. This skill benefits students across all subjects, from math to art.
- **Supports critical thinking and problem-solving:** Skills such as understanding cause-and-effect relationships and making predictions are key components of critical thinking. These skills are also extremely language based. By working on these skills, students are better equipped to analyze information, draw conclusions, and solve problems. These abilities are central to subjects like science and social studies.

- **Increases participation in class discussions:** Strengthening expressive language skills allows students to express their thoughts and ideas, ask questions, and engage in classroom discussions. This participation fosters deeper understanding of the curriculum content. This skill can be beneficial in subjects that involve group work or presentations.
- **Builds written expression skills:** Language skills directly impact students' ability to organize and express their ideas in writing. Improved sentence structure and vocabulary help students create coherent essays, reports, and responses to prompts, which are essential for success in both language arts, social studies, and any subject that requires written expression. Standardized tests that students must take in school often require written responses as well.

THE PROBLEM WITH STICKING TO THE CURRICULUM

Besides the fact that the curriculum is often too challenging and boring for these students, there are other problems you might face when you are trying to use the curriculum to plan your sessions. The following list breaks down these challenges:

- **Scheduling challenges**: Often, you'll have students who are coming from different classes, different grades, or the classes are working on different topics at the same time. It can be a challenge to find one unit they are all working on together.
- **You are in the dark:** No matter how hard you try, you might not always get updates from the classroom teachers about what they are working on. You can use curriculum maps and guides, but it doesn't always tell you exactly where they are individually. You can ask your students what they are working on or struggling with but that often leads to blank stares or insufficient details.
- **It is a juggling act:** Even if you get updates and details from teachers or students, it can be a challenge to prepare in time for the sessions or have enough time to work with all students with what they need in the moment. There are only so many hours in a day.
- **Ensuring carry-over:** You can help students with essays and vocabulary. You can help them study for tests. But are you working on the root cause of their struggle? Are you teaching them how to make progress on their goals when you are not there? Is this ensuring carry-over?
- **You feel like a tutor:** When you are just helping your students study or complete homework, you might wonder about your role and question whether you are truly working on speech and language skills. You can fall into the trap of just helping them with their work and neglecting the skills they truly need to be working on.

WHY READING LEVELS MATTER MORE THAN GRADE LEVELS

To be an effective and skilled reader, a student needs adequate language comprehension skills. Speech and language students are often reading below or even way below their grade level. They are often falling farther and farther behind their peers and are constantly presented with material that is too challenging for them. When we also present them with material like this, they can shut down, avoid, or just be frustrated. Handing a struggling reader a Shakespearean sonnet and expecting them to thrive is like giving someone a smartphone in airplane mode and asking them to Google the solution. It's not happening.

On the other hand, when you provide your students with content that is at their independent reading level, you are setting them up for success. Their independent reading level indicates what they can read without assistance. You can determine this in several ways:

- Ask a teacher or reading specialist who might have that information.
- Look at their educational testing results as part of their IEP process. It may indicate a grade level equivalent or some sort of informal notation on a report or in the present level of performance section on an IEP.
- Probe yourself to see where they are the most comfortable.

TIP

I provide a digital critical thinking probing tool on my free resources page that comes with this book. This tool helps you determine which reading level is appropriate for your individual student from three different reading levels and what length the student performs optimally at as well. It provides various multiple choice questions to assess how they perform at tasks, such as main ideas, making inferences, and using context clues. Visit www.speechtimefun.com/book to grab this free informal assessment tool.

I will never forget the moment when I realized the value of using appropriate levels with my students. I was working with a fifth-grade boy. We were reading an article about the history of YouTube to work on note-taking and responding to inferential questions, and he kept requesting to read. At one point, he stopped and said, "I don't like to read in class, but I like to read in here." It made me stop and reflect on why that might be. In class he was expected to read challenging texts that he didn't feel comfortable reading, especially out loud in front of his peers. But he recognized that I provided him with texts that he could decode with ease and feel confident reading in front of his peers.

If using a simplified text can lead to more participation, more confidence, and more progress, why wouldn't we use one? Get those quick wins first. Show students that they can succeed. SLPs have the flexibility to use whatever materials we want, so why not use what will actually work?

FINDING AGE-APPROPRIATE RESOURCES

It can be a challenge to find resources that are at simplified reading levels yet don't look like they are designed for younger students. Just because they are reading at a first- or second-grade level, doesn't mean you are going to provide a middle schooler with a worksheet designed for a first or second grader.

Here's a list of resources where you can find simplified texts for students reading below grade level:

- **Newsela:** This site offers leveled news articles on current events and topics, with content adapted to various reading levels. You can take one article and change the Lexile to meet the needs of your students with a click of a button. You can get access to some texts with a free subscription or access to more with a paid one. Many school districts have access to this site, and you can request access.
- **ReadWorks**: This site provides free, leveled reading passages and question sets. It has options to filter by grade and reading level. You can also search and find passages based on language comprehension skills you are trying to address. Although you cannot change the Lexile of a passage you find, you can search by reading levels.
- **CommonLit**: This site includes a wide range of texts with different reading levels, comprehension questions, and additional supports for struggling readers. You can register for a free educator account.
- **Storyworks (Scholastic)**: This is a subscription service that offers differentiated reading material, including fiction, nonfiction, and poetry for various reading levels.
- **Epic!**: This is a digital library with thousands of books sorted by age and reading level, including options for struggling readers. You can access a free account with an educator email address.

- **Tar Heel Reader**: Also known now as the Monarch Reader, this site provides a collection of free, accessible books designed for students with diverse learning needs and lower reading levels.
- **Oxford Owl**: This website has free ebooks and reading resources at different levels, focusing on early readers and struggling readers. You need to register for a free account by entering the school that you work for. You can also get access to a parent account for free resources as well.
- **Raz-Kids (Learning A-Z)**: This is a subscription-based resource with leveled books that include audio support, quizzes, and other reading aids.
- **DOGO News**: This website offers articles on high interest topics. It provides real photos and video clips related to the articles which helps with background knowledge and understanding. It provides reading levels, texts in English and Spanish, the ability to listen to the text, and games to learn the keywords or vocabulary included in the text. With a paid subscription, you can toggle to simplify the text.
- **SLP Elevate**: Of course I had to include my subscription option which provides brand-new articles every month related to a new high-interest theme. Every month members get access to six new articles, fiction and nonfiction, and various reading levels. They also get access to task card games for those needing more at the paragraph level. It also provides access to picture stories for those needing even more support.

A Game-Changer: Using AI to Adapt Materials

This section would not be complete if I did not share about an artificial intelligence tool for educators. Diffit for teachers (see https://app.diffit.me/) is a tool that just requires an email login. You can search for "literally everything," as the site states. You can search for various topics, subjects, and grade levels.

My favorite feature is that you can enter the URL of a website and customize the reading level on that site. That means you can take an article on DOGO News and simplify it yourself. You can even take sites that do not have various reading level options, like TweenTribune, and customize them to meet your needs. You can also paste from a text or upload a PDF file to customize as well. You can even type in a passage from a novel or textbook your students are reading in class and adapt it to meet their needs.

Diffit makes it simple to modify and adapt the classroom resource so students can access the curriculum. It will even generate images from a text, provide a summary, pull key vocabulary and definitions, and generate comprehension questions with multiple choice answers. With the click of a button, you can generate student activities and materials. With access to a tool like this, you can no longer say that you cannot find materials at simplified reading levels or that you wish an article you found was simplified. This site really is amazing and a game changer. If you have not played around with it, go put a bookmark in right now and go play! I promise you will be amazed.

Age-Appropriate Versus Age-Respectful

When choosing materials for older students, especially those reading below grade level, it is important to understand the difference between *age-appropriate* and *age-respectful* resources.

Age-appropriate materials match a student's chronological age in terms of topic and theme. So for a teenager, that might mean books or articles about high school life, relationships, social media, or pop culture. But here's the catch: just because a material is age-appropriate doesn't mean it is accessible. A high schooler who is reading at a third-grade reading level might be interested in those topics but will struggle to read a text if it is written at a high school level. That mismatch can leave students feeling discouraged or overwhelmed. These students often avoid reading tasks all together.

That is where age-respectful materials come in. These are designed to honor the student's age and maturity level, while being readable and understandable based on their language and reading skills. The themes are still relevant to them (e.g., friendship, anime, getting a job), but the vocabulary, sentence structure, and overall complexity is scaled down. Age-respectful materials give students access to content that feels appropriate for their stage of life, without making them feel like it is too "childlike" or hard to follow.

I remember working with a tenth-grade student who loved Pokémon. On the surface, that might seem too young for a high schooler, and I caught myself wondering if I should steer him toward something else. But rather than dismissing his interest, I decided to lean into it. We started using Pokémon-themed materials to work on narrative structure and describing character traits. I even found an article that was written at a fifth-grade level that compared Pokémon types to animal groups in biology (which was what he was working on in science class) and he was hooked. It showed me what was possible when I used a student's interests to challenge them in an age-respectful way.

You might be thinking, "But what if my student is older and still loves things that seem more juvenile?" That is a common challenge, and the good news is that you don't have to completely avoid those interests. If a student loves SpongeBob, that doesn't mean that you are stuck using babyish materials. That also doesn't mean you avoid their interests and try to convince them to like other things. You can use characters and scenes from the show to explore age-respectful concepts, like how to solve problems or handle conflicts. You can also pull out themes and connect them to more neutral or mature content. For example, you can use Sponge-Bob's obsession with Krabby Patties to transition to a discussion about burgers or even getting a job at a burger place.

The big takeaway here is that age-appropriate materials reflect the student's age in terms of topic but may not meet them where they are academically. Age-respectful materials strike a balance. They respect the student's maturity and social world while adjusting the complexity so that students can engage and succeed.

A Simple Tweak to Show How Language Activities Are Relevant

So how do you take these isolated language activities and make them relevant to the classroom? Teachers are often working on these skills in the classroom, so it is relevant. Students are expected to respond to inferential questions, write summaries, make predictions, and more in the classroom. The way you introduce and conclude a session can help students see how this approach can help them in the classroom.

An introduction to a lesson doesn't need to be elaborate or drawn out. It could take seconds or a few minutes. But explaining to your students what you will be working on and how it will help them can go a long way. For example, if you are working on expressing main ideas, you can say, "Has your teacher ever asked you 'what is this story all about?' It can be difficult to know exactly what to say. Do you say everything? A few sentences? One word? And why are they asking you that anyway? Well, they are asking you about the main idea which can show them that you understand what was just read in a simple sentence. I am going to show you a way to make it super simple so that you know exactly what to say." By starting out the session by building the stage for what you are doing and how it is relevant to them, it will get their buy-in and show them that what you are doing isn't arbitrary or random.

A conclusion to a session is also important to show your students how this approach is relevant and how they now have a skill that they can generalize outside of your speech room. It also doesn't need to be elaborate or take a long time. Using the previous example, "So, when your teacher asks you what the story was all about, how will you respond?" Taking the time to review this at the end of the session is also a great way to build their confidence and show them what they accomplished in that 30-minute speech session.

Incorporating an introduction and conclusion to your session is a great for building a routine. It helps you remember to always do it, but it also helps students always know that it is being provided and that what you are doing is always relevant. You don't need to know what they are working on in science or math to be able to do this. You don't need to be an expert on the curriculum to know that teachers may ask questions like this in various subjects. You know they need to follow directions and read complex sentences in math. You know they need to make hypotheses, follow directions, understand cause/effect, and make predictions in science. You know social studies requires understanding sequence of events, being able to describe events in history, and even compare/contrast. You know that in English language arts students are expected to answer various comprehension question types. You can use this basic knowledge to build introductions and conclusions.

REAL RESULTS: SHIFTING AWAY FROM CURRICULUM-BASED LESSONS

One of the most common challenges that SLPs face is the pressure to adapt grade-level curriculum to their students' needs. It can feel like the logical solution—taking what the classroom teacher is using and modifying it to fit speech and language goals. But as many SLPs discover, this approach often leads to frustration and inefficiency.

Thoughts From the Field

SLP Elevate member Sandra Clausen used to struggle with this. She shared with me how this mindset was holding her back. At first, she thought adapting resources meant using grade-level content and creating separate activities for each grade to target specific student goals. She was spending hours trying to tailor materials for each grade, but it rarely worked out the way she had hoped. She felt incompetent.

"Hallie has helped me realize that adapting resources doesn't mean using each grade levels' content and creating activities with each separate content to target student goals. I was putting so much work into each grade levels' content. Some of my activities were a hit for some students, but they were never perfect for all students, and when an activity that I spent an hour on was a bust, I felt incompetent. Hallie helped me release needing eight different topics for middle

(continued)

(continued)

and high school students and target skill building more. I'm finally able to spend more time on strategies, facilitating neurological affirming interventions, collaboration, and special projects. It is so terrific having Hallie's community behind me. I've gotten support in meeting the needs of students using AAC and fantastic materials each month that deep-dive skill-building with a variety of goal types, not just a few!!"

Using curriculum-based materials often sets both the student and the SLP up for failure. Grade-level content assumes students are already operating at a level they're not yet ready for. It often leads to activities that are either too difficult, resulting in avoidance behaviors, or so simplified that they feel "babyish" and disengaging.

When you instead choose materials that align with a student's actual abilities, you can meet them where they are and build the skills they truly need. This not only leads to more student success but also allows you to feel more effective and confident in your role.

The Goldilocks Rule

You should now have a better understanding of why speech and language students need materials at their own levels so that they can access the curriculum. You want your lessons to feel relevant, functional, and fun. You want your students to enjoy participating, not feel forced to do so. You want them to see the benefits to the class.

It is the Goldilocks Rule: The activities and materials should not be so easy that students think they are juvenile and not worth their time. But you also don't want them to be so challenging that students shut down. You need them to be just right.

You can do this without the curriculum. You can use materials that help you address their language goals in isolation and then show them how to apply it to what they are doing in the classroom. Think of it like adjusting the thermostat: too hot (challenging) and they'll burn out; too cold (easy) and they'll check out. You're aiming for that "just right" zone where learning feels achievable and rewarding.

NOW WHAT?

If you have not already played around and checked out all the sites and tools I shared in this chapter, go ahead and see what is available. Can you find some articles that incorporate your students' interests? Can you find materials at your students' reading levels? The more tools you have, the more prepared you'll feel, and the more equipped you will be to handle students' needs.

I encourage you to take some time to reflect and think about these questions:

- What has been your experience with using curriculum-based materials in speech therapy?
  - Did you feel they were effective?
  - How did your students respond to them?
- How do you currently choose materials for your sessions?
  - Are you prioritizing reading levels, interests, or goals?
  - What adjustments could you make to improve relevance and engagement?
- Have you noticed any patterns in your students' participation or motivation?
  - When are they most engaged?
  - What factors (e.g., difficulty level, topic) contribute to their engagement?
- Are you effectively showing your students how their speech work translates to classroom success?
  - How often do you introduce and conclude sessions with a clear connection to their classroom experience?
- What tools or resources are you currently using, and how well are they working?
  - Do you feel limited by available materials?
  - Have you explored resources like Newsela, Diffit, or SLP Elevate?

Here are some steps you can take right away to put what you have learned in this chapter into action:

- Identify your students' needs:
  - Select one or two students to start with.
  - Determine their independent reading levels using available tools or probes.
  - Review their IEP goals to ensure materials and activities align with their needs.
- Explore new resources:
  - Choose at least one new resource (e.g., Newsela, Diffit, ReadWorks) and experiment with adapting materials for a current student or group.
  - Bookmark your favorite resource for quick access in future planning sessions.

- Practice the "introduction and conclusion" strategy:
  - Write down how you'll introduce the relevance of the next session's skill to the classroom or in real life.
  - Script a brief conclusion that highlights how the skill can help your students outside of the speech room.
- Start small with age-respectful materials:
  - Select one simplified, age-respectful text or activity to test with a group.
  - Observe how students respond and adapt as needed for future sessions.
- Reflect and adjust:
  - After your next session, take five minutes to reflect on what worked well and what could be improved.
  - Use this reflection to tweak your approach for the next session.
- Get feedback:
  - Ask your students for feedback on a recent session: "Did this lesson help you with something in class?" or "What did you like about today's activity?"
  - Use their input to refine your methods and materials.

The next chapter talks about adapting resources. It explains in more detail how to take one activity and use it with as many groups as possible. I cannot wait to share this with you!

CHAPTER 11

Adapting Resources and Using Fewer Materials

Let's go way back in time to the early days of Hallie the SLP. I planned a unique lesson, with unique materials, for every session of the day. I remember frantically preparing individual lessons late into the night, convinced that each student needed a completely unique plan to succeed. My desk was a sea of sticky notes, file folders, and half-finished ideas, but I still felt like I was barely staying afloat. Every student had different goals, and I found a different game, book, article, or activity for each group. I had a cute planner I found online that I used to document what I was doing for every session. I created file folders, labeled them for every group, and placed worksheets in each one that I could pull from. I felt so organized and prepared. I had a ton of resources to pull from. Each group came, I pulled the worksheet from the folder or grabbed the game off the shelf. They left, I cleaned it up and grabbed what I needed for the next group. I did not know any different. I learned from graduate school to plan for every goal and every session.

Although I had things ready to go and felt prepared, I was spending all my preparation period, which I was fortunate to have, deciding what to work on, finding resources, and filling my file folders. The problem with this was that I did not have time left for other aspects of my job such as report writing, calling parents, and preparing for meetings. I did not have time in between sessions to reflect on what worked and what did not work since I had to prepare for the next session. I was not taking the time to even truly understand what I was working on or how I was teaching it. I was just finding "stuff" to get the job done. I wasn't excited about my activities because they weren't that exciting. I wasn't taking the time to teach the skills; we were just practicing.

As my caseload grew, my piles of "stuff" grew, and I realized I could not go on like that. It was not effective. I realized I was experiencing materials overwhelm. I felt buried under the sheer volume of resources, tools, and materials I thought that I needed to use or create. This created stress, confusion, and a feeling of inefficiency.

Maybe you have felt this way. Materials overwhelm is like trying to pack for a trip with a suitcase that's already overflowing. Every time you add another item, it feels necessary and specific for the trip, but soon you're so buried in clothing, gadgets, and "just-in-case" items that you can barely close the suitcase. Instead of feeling ready and organized, you end up feeling weighed down, unsure of where everything is, and worried you might have forgotten something essential.

PREVENTING MATERIALS OVERWHELM

For school-based SLPs, materials overwhelm can occur when they attempt to prepare unique materials for every single therapy session. While it's natural to want customized resources to meet each student's needs, constantly creating new materials can lead to burnout. It takes up time that could otherwise be spent engaging with students or working on professional development, and it can make therapy planning seem like a never-ending task.

Here are some strategies to help manage this potential overwhelm:

- **Standardize and reuse materials:** Develop a set of versatile, go-to materials that can be easily adapted to different goals or students. Instead of creating a new worksheet or activity for each session, find materials that can be modified on the fly.
- **Batch create and organize:** Set aside dedicated time to create or organize materials for commonly targeted goals (e.g., articulation, language comprehension, social skills) rather than doing this weekly or daily. Create a system that makes it easy to grab what you need quickly. Whether it is a filing cabinet or plastic bins, having dedicated spots for your materials makes it easy to grab and go. I also love having my most used graphic organizers in magnetic folders near my therapy table so that I can easily grab them as needed. I make multiple photocopies and have always them on hand.

> **TIP**
>
> You can see this storage on my Instagram at www.instagram.com/p/DAMhArfMBDE/.

- **Digital resources and templates:** Consider using digital resources or templates that can be reused and adapted without requiring physical storage. Google Slides and Boom Card activities are a great way to reduce the need for paper materials that take of a lot of space. There are tons of premade materials online that can also reduce prep time.

- **Delegate materials creation to students (when appropriate):** Older students can be part of the materials-prep process. They can help create flashcards or other materials, which not only reduces your workload but also engages them in the learning process.
- **Set realistic goals for each session:** Remember that less is often more. Focus on a single target skill or goal rather than trying to address multiple objectives in each session. This helps streamline your materials. You only have your students for 20–30 minutes. They each have different goals and needs. You cannot work on everything. If you try to work on everything, you will work on nothing.

By setting up some of these strategies, you can reduce the pressure to be constantly creating, which can alleviate stress and allow you to focus more on the quality of therapy rather than the quantity of materials.

DIVING DEEPER INTO BATCH PLANNING

Batch planning is a powerful strategy to streamline your preparation process, reduce stress, and reclaim your time. Instead of planning each session or group individually as they come up, you dedicate a focused block of time to prepare materials and resources that can be used across multiple sessions, groups, or goals. Think of it as meal prepping for your therapy sessions—investing a little time up front saves you countless hours later.

Wondering if batch planning is for your or if it will really work? Here are some of the benefits of batch planning:

- **Efficiency:** When you're in "creation mode," you can prepare multiple materials more quickly than switching between planning, therapy, and administrative tasks.
- **Consistency:** By creating materials in bulk, you ensure a cohesive approach to your sessions and avoid scrambling for resources at the last minute.
- **Reduced Stress:** Knowing you have ready-to-go materials for several weeks or even months allows you to focus on engaging with your students instead of juggling endless preparation.
- **Flexibility:** By batching versatile materials, you can adapt them on the fly to meet various student needs without feeling unprepared.

Implementing Batch Planning

Try these steps to implement batch planning:

1. **Identify common goals**
   - Start by analyzing your caseload and grouping similar goals. For example, if many of your students are working on main idea, articulation, or social skills, prioritize creating resources that target these areas.
   - Example: If you have three groups working on comprehension skills, you can prepare materials like short texts, graphic organizers, and comprehension question prompts that can be reused across groups.

2. **Choose a dedicated time**
   - Set aside a specific block of time weekly, biweekly, or monthly for batch planning. Treat it like an appointment you can't skip.
   - Example: Friday afternoons could be your planning day, where you create resources for the following two weeks.

3. **Use themes to maximize impact**
   - Create materials based on high-interest themes or topics that can be applied across multiple groups. For instance, a theme like "superheroes" could include articles, vocabulary games, and discussion prompts.
   - Example: Prepare superhero-themed materials that address articulation (e.g., target sounds in superhero names), comprehension (e.g., main idea in superhero articles), and social skills (e.g., role-playing scenarios based on superhero teamwork).

4. **Prepare multigoal resources**
   - Focus on materials that can target a variety of goals. For example:
     - Articles with comprehension questions for language goals
     - Picture prompts for articulation and inferencing
     - Videos or interactive games that work for both social skills and critical thinking
   - Example: Create a YouTube video guide for students to practice summarizing, retelling, answering WH questions, and observing social interactions.

5. **Organize your materials**
   - Create an efficient storage system for easy access. Use labeled bins, digital folders, or color-coded binders to keep materials sorted by goal, age group, or theme.
   - Example: Dedicate one binder to articulation, another to comprehension, and another to social skills. Use dividers for specific subgoals (e.g., /s/ sounds or inferencing).

6. **Incorporate digital tools**
   - Use platforms like Google Drive, Boom Cards, or Teachers Pay Teachers to organize and store digital resources. These tools allow you to easily tweak and reuse materials without needing physical storage. SLP Elevate organizes resources for you by theme and by goal/skill.
   - Example: Create a Google Drive folder with subfolders for themes or goals, and upload PDFs, slideshows, and cheat sheets for quick access.
7. **Automate repetitive tasks**
   - Use templates for commonly needed materials like data sheets, evaluation forms, or visual aids. Save time by modifying these templates instead of starting from scratch.
   - Example: Use a main idea graphic organizer template that you can fill in with new content each week.

Example Batch Planning Session

Let's say you set aside one to two hours on a Friday afternoon for batch planning. Here's how you could structure your time:

1. **Identify goals (15 minutes):** Review your caseload and prioritize common goals for the next two weeks (e.g., main idea, articulation of /r/, inferencing).
2. **Choose materials (45 minutes):** Select two to three versatile resources (e.g., a short article, a set of picture cards, and a Jeopardy game) and decide how to adapt them for multiple goals.
3. **Prepare and print (30 minutes):** Create cheat sheets, print graphic organizers, and label materials for easy access. Save digital resources in an organized folder for quick use.
4. **Organize (20 minutes):** File printed materials in labeled folders or bins. Update your planner with a list of activities for each group and goal.

Batch Planning in Action

Here's how batch planning might look for a comprehension goal:

Week Theme: Winter Sports

- Find an article (e.g., from Newsela, ReadWorks, or SLP Elevate).
- Create comprehension questions for language goals (with SLP Elevate you get access to those questions).

- Highlight target articulation sounds in the text (note that with SLP Elevate you also get access to supplemental articulation activities related to the theme).
- Develop a social skills activity based on teamwork in sports (with SLP Elevate you get access to social skills activities related to the theme and articles).

TIP

With SLP Elevate, since you get access to the articles, comprehension questions, and supplemental activities, you can easily cut the time from one to two hours to prep for the week to less than one hour! Visit www.slpelevate.com to find out more.

USING VERSATILE MATERIALS

SLPs love materials. They can be hoarders at times. However, I have found it to be much easier and less overwhelming to have fewer materials that can be used across multiple goals and purposes. Using one activity for only one goal is like using a Swiss Army knife to only open a can and ignoring all the other tools it has. It's functional, but you're missing out on its full potential. In contrast, using that same activity to target multiple goals is like fully utilizing the Swiss Army knife: you can open a can, cut a rope, file down a rough edge, and screw in a bolt—all with the same tool. Similarly, when you adapt one activity to work on multiple goals, you're maximizing its utility, saving time, and meeting diverse needs with a single, flexible resource.

Here are some versatile materials that can be incredibly useful for targeting multiple goals with secondary speech students and examples of different goals you can use with them:

- **Picture cards or scene cards:** Use cards with images depicting scenes, objects, or actions. These can work for articulation (practicing sounds within descriptions), language goals (building sentences, describing, inferencing), and social-pragmatic skills (interpreting scenes, discussing emotions, creating conversation starters).

TIP

You can find these cards on Teachers Pay Teachers, on SLP Elevate with membership, or even just use Google Images or the *New York Times'* "What's Going on in This Picture?" https://www.nytimes.com/column/learning-whats-going-on-in-this-picture.

- **Text-based prompts (e.g., news articles, short stories, or paragraphs):** Short texts are excellent for practicing reading comprehension, vocabulary, inferencing, summarizing, and articulation when students read aloud. These can also spark discussions for pragmatic language and social interaction skills. I shared in the previous chapter my favorite spots to grab articles and text-based activities. Find ones that incorporate students' interests and are at their reading levels. Provide follow-up activities to meet the various needs and goals.
- **Dry erase board and markers:** A simple dry erase board can be used for drawing or mapping out concepts, practicing written language goals, building vocabulary through word webs, illustrating social scenarios, or practicing articulation by writing out words or sentences with target sounds. Students love dry erase so why not use it for various purposes?
- **Graphic organizers:** These can be applied to many goals, such as organizing thoughts before speaking, creating summaries of what was read or heard, mapping out story elements, and working on social scenarios. Graphic organizers can also be personalized to fit individual needs without having to create something entirely new for each session.
- **Games with open-ended questions (e.g., Jenga, Uno, Connect Four with question cards):** You can attach questions or prompts to each turn in the game, like answering a comprehension question, practicing a sound, or discussing a social scenario. These games are engaging and adaptable to most therapy goals, adding a fun and motivating aspect to the sessions. You can create a "key" for different colors of a game to indicate different tasks a student has to do when they pull that color, and every student can get a different key based on their goals.

TIP

You can see an example of this on my Instagram at www.instagram.com/p/DA50CMLtWOZ/?img_index=1.

- **Dice:** Dice can turn anything into a game. Students can roll to determine how many times they need to practice their articulation sound, to get points for answering a question on a worksheet correctly, to determine how many items in a category they must name, and so much more.

TIP

You can find digital dice on Toy Theater. They have multiple dice options, even ones with higher numbers. Check it out at https://toytheater.com/dice/.

- **Books:** Just like with text-based articles, you can do the same with books. Many storybooks are written at a fifth-grade reading level, but you can also use wordless picture books and graphic novels. You can work on summarizing, answering questions, building vocabulary, and even retelling using articulation targets.
- **Song lyrics:** Students love music and there are so many free song lyrics available online that you can print and use. Students can work on vocabulary, perspective taking, sentence structure, verb tenses, comprehension, and more. You can even reward them at the end by playing karaoke.
- **Jokes:** You can find free jokes for kids online. Jokes are embedded with a ton of language such as figurative language and multiple-meaning words, and students struggle to understand the humor. t You can also find jokes that are bombarded with their articulation sound. You can role-play telling jokes in different social scenarios. The possibilities are endless.
- **YouTube Videos:** I love using YouTube with my students. It is fun but it is also easy to adapt to meet various goals. With one video, you can work on retelling, answering questions, retelling with articulation targets, body language and social skills, main idea, and so much more.

> ## TIP
>
> I included samples of my YouTube Cheat Sheets on my resource page so you can try two different videos that have a variety of goals and prompts you can use. Just print out the cheat sheets, open YouTube, and have fun! Head to www.speechtimefun.com/book to access this free resource.

These versatile materials help streamline planning and help you prevent materials overwhelm. You don't need a lot of stuff, but you do need to be open-minded and willing to look at an activity or resource and see all the possibilities you can do with it. Just change your questioning, change your objective, change the way you teach it, but use the same materials with as many groups and goals as possible to save yourself time and energy.

Benefits of Adapting Resources

There are so many benefits to adapting resources. Here are three key benefits:

- **Efficiency and time savings:** By using materials that can serve multiple purposes, you reduce the need to create or prepare new resources for every individual goal. This streamlines your planning process, giving you more time to focus on engaging with students and tailoring instruction to their needs rather than getting bogged down in prep work. Plus, it gives you more time to do the other aspects of your job like billing, writing IEPs, and so on. Imagine freeing up 20 minutes every day—enough for that second cup of coffee or tackling overdue paperwork!

- **Increased student engagement:** Versatile materials often lend themselves to creative and dynamic use, which can make sessions more engaging for students. By adapting activities to fit multiple goals, you can keep things fresh without constantly introducing new materials. Students enjoy the variety and familiarity, allowing them to focus on learning rather than adjusting to new activities each session. Plus, you can have all students working together in a session and engage with each other.
- **Consistency and skill generalization:** Reusing familiar materials across goals allows students to see connections between skills and apply them across contexts. For example, working on articulation within a comprehension activity helps students practice sounds while understanding language, which promotes generalization and helps them transfer skills more naturally into real-life communication situations.

Risks of Adapting Resources

While adapting resources for multiple goals has many benefits and is something I highly recommend, there are potential risks to be aware of:

- **Dilution of a specific skill focus:** When a single resource is adapted for various goals, it's possible that the primary focus may become less clear. For instance, using one activity to target both articulation and language comprehension might mean that one of these goals doesn't get the intensity it needs. It's essential to maintain clear objectives for each goal, even within a versatile resource. Make sure you are constantly expressing the objectives for each goal and students are aware of what they are individually working on.
- **Overwhelming students:** If a resource is stretched to cover too many goals at once, students might feel confused or overwhelmed by the shifting expectations within a single activity. This is especially a concern for students who benefit from clear, singular focus or struggle with multitasking. Ensuring that instructions and objectives are clear is key to managing this. Again, this is also why it is important for students to be focusing on only one goal per session, even if they have multiple goals to work on.

- **Difficulty tracking progress:** Adapting one resource for multiple goals may make it challenging to isolate progress in individual areas. Without focused, goal-specific activities, it could be harder to measure growth in each skill area accurately. Adding checkpoints or specific observation notes can help mitigate this risk and provide clarity in progress tracking. I cover data collection in more depth in Chapter 12 about working with mixed groups.

By being aware of these risks, you can take steps to ensure that adapted resources remain effective and focused on student progress. This isn't to make you worried or concerned about using fewer materials or adapting materials, but to just be mindful of what could go wrong and how to prevent it from happening.

Using Materials Beyond How They Are Intended

I shared several ways to adapt resources to meet the various needs of your students. But you can also take things you have, that you may have found online for a specific goal and use it for other goals. This allows you to have more opportunities to use the activity and plan with less stuff. Imagine using a single article about YouTube history: for comprehension, students summarize the main idea; for articulation, they practice target sounds in specific words from the text; for social skills, they role-play discussing the article with a peer.

Let's say you found a task card game or activity to work on main idea with paragraphs. You can use that to work on other goals. You can have students summarize the paragraphs, you can ask WH questions, and you can even ask inferential questions based on those paragraphs. You can pull the paragraphs that are bombarded with an articulation target and use it for an articulation activity.

> **TIP**
>
> Here is a real example you can use. The Jeopardy game on JeopardyLabs.com is for expressing a main idea. Just copy and paste this link into a browser to play this free game: https://jeopardylabs.com/play/main-idea-for-each-passage-state-the-main-idea-12. You can use this game for more than just main idea. Ask a different question. Work on summarizing, inferential questions, recalling details, and more. The sky is the limit when you think outside the box.

NOW WHAT?

In this chapter, I shared the benefits of using fewer materials and the problems you can face by using too many materials. I shared several examples of how you can use the materials that you have to target a variety of speech and language goals. I even shared sample games and sites for you to access free materials to try this out. I hope you found it helpful to see real examples and even got to check some things out. This approach can help you when working with any age group in a school setting. It doesn't just apply to secondary students. I find it is even easier with secondary students when so many of them have comprehension goals. I also find that SLPs working with secondary students tend to have larger caseloads, mixed groups, and are in multiple buildings, all of which make it even more necessary to work smarter not harder.

Go peek at what you have. Maybe some books on your bookshelf. Look at some of the text-based suggestions I provided. Think of how many goals you can address. What would you need to add to it to get the job done? A graphic organizer? A visual? Maybe a cheat sheet of different prompts to make sure you have them to cover the various goals? Grab the free YouTube cheat sheets as well. My hope is that you start looking at activities differently. Instead of looking for materials for specific goals, look at activities and wonder how many goals can be targeted with it. The more goals, the better! There are no limits. Remember, you can use activities to work on different goals than they were intended for. Your students won't notice or care.

By rethinking how you use your materials, you can transform your sessions into efficient, impactful experiences—for you and your students. Start small, experiment, and trust your instincts. You've got this!

Go take some action!

- Spend 15 minutes this week identifying two to three versatile resources you already have. Brainstorm how to adapt them for multiple goals.
- Choose one group session to test using a single resource for diverse goals. Observe how it changes engagement and progress tracking.

12

Mixed Groups Made Easy

As a new SLP, I was shocked to see so many different goals in one group. Five students with different needs, and only 30 minutes to address it all. Students with articulation, social skills, and language needs were all in one group together. How in the world was I going to do this? I also inherited students with many goals to accomplish in one year. Sixty-five students on a caseload, each with three to five goals. I was only working with them once or twice a week. I was overwhelmed and unsure.

I did not want anyone to know that I was unsure of myself. I did not want to appear inadequate. I tried everything. I worked with each student individually to make sure their needs were met. I did not have a large enough therapy space for stations, but I researched this possibility. With stations, some students work independently while others work with the SLP. The problem with working individually with students was that each student was waiting around, bored, while I worked with the others, and I was planning five different activities for one session. I felt rushed, frazzled, and inefficient. I tried making smaller groups with fewer students working on different things. I had too many groups and not enough hours in a day. I still needed a ton of materials and activities to meet all their needs, and I did not have a second to breathe in between sessions. I started to mix up activities, using the wrong activity with the wrong group, doing the same activity twice with a group, and so many other mistakes.

I realized I needed to work smarter and not harder. I needed to take one activity and make it work for all. Once I started doing that, I had students working together, learning from each other, and requiring fewer activities and materials. The more I started doing this, the more I was able to take any activity and adapt it to meet all the needs of the group. I was then able to plan in minutes. Students were all participating and not waiting around. I felt less frazzled and overwhelmed. I felt more efficient. I did not fear larger groups and was able to see fewer groups in a day. I also realized that less is more with goals and started to write IEPs with fewer yearly goals.

THE MIXED-GROUP CHALLENGE

Whether you like it or not, you must deal with mixed groups. Especially with older students that come to speech less often and have less availability in their schedules, you must pull students when you can. Some students may come during lunch, others can only come during specials like home economics or art. You have students working on different goals in a group. Instead of fearing these groups, it's time to embrace them.

Why do many SLPs dislike these groups? It is hard! An SLP working with a mixed speech and language group is like a chef orchestrating a multicourse meal with different dishes for every guest. Just like our students with individual speech and language goals, imagine each of these guests have unique dietary needs. One guest needs the spices added just right, another has food allergies, while a third needs the food at a specific temperature. The chef must balance all the plates, adjusting ingredients and pacing to serve each customer exactly what they need. They need to do this to keep the kitchen running smoothly while making sure no one leaves hungry for progress. Just like the chef juggling it all, we must juggle it all to have our speech rooms run smoothly.

The problem with working individually in a group setting is that you cannot utilize the entire session for an individual student. Assume that you have a group of five students for 30 minutes. If you are working individually with each, you are only giving each student 20% of your attention. That is only six minutes of attention and instruction. With the least restrictive environment, you are encouraged to keep students in their general education setting as much as possible. If you are pulling them out of class to sit around for 24 minutes, is that the best use of their time? Even if you are doing stations and having them practice independently, couldn't they do that in the classroom or for home practice?

SHIFTING SOME BELIEFS

As SLPs, we pick up a lot of beliefs throughout our training and careers. Some are explicitly taught, while others are simply absorbed along the way. These beliefs often shape how we view things like mixed groups. Let's be honest, mixed groups are not ideal, are overwhelming, and can even be frustrating. Over time, I have found that reframing some of the ideas I had about mixed groups has completely changed the way I approached them. They became more doable and even enjoyable.

One of the biggest mindset shifts for me was moving away from the idea that more trials always equal better results. I used to think that if I didn't hit a certain number of trials, the session wasn't "successful." But I've learned that quality matters so much more than quantity. One supported trial with meaningful feedback can do more for a student than ten rushed ones. It can be a challenge to get enough trials in a mixed group, but it is more beneficial that students learn from each other.

Another belief I had to let go of was that students needed one-on-one time to make meaningful progress. In reality, I've seen some of the biggest breakthroughs happen in group settings. Mixed groups allow for peer modeling, natural turn-taking, and real-time social interaction. I had a group once where a student suddenly started using more complex sentences. It wasn't because of something that I said, but because she wanted to match what another student in the group was doing. That kind of peer influence can be powerful and something we should lean into rather than fear.

Speaking of peers, I used to worry that students couldn't really learn from each other. I thought it was all on me to lead the instruction. But over and over again, I've seen how students can rise to the occasion when given the chance. They echo each other's strategies, celebrate wins, and sometimes explain things in a way that clicks better than I ever could.

Another shift came when I stopped trying to plan individualized activities for every single student in the group. I used to run myself ragged prepping five different activities for five different goals I needed to address for a session. But I have found that a single, well-chosen activity can touch upon multiple goals if you are strategic. A shared storybook, for example, might be used to practice articulation for one student, vocabulary with another, and sentence construction or social skills with the rest. It takes some practice, but designing with flexibility in mind has saved me so much time and mental energy. It also brings a sense of cohesion to the group.

And finally, maybe the biggest shift of them all: the belief that mixed groups are inherently chaotic or unmanageable. I used to go into the session bracing for a storm. But once I leaned into structure with clear routines and flexible materials, I felt so much more in control. The students knew what to expect, and that predictability created space for real learning and fun. I wasn't reacting to the chaos; I was leading with intention.

All of this to say that the way you think about trials, individualization, and peer dynamics matters. Mixed groups don't have to be a source for stress. With a few mindset shifts, they can become a space for potential. It can be a space for connection, growth, and meaningful progress. It isn't about doing more, but about doing things differently, and in a way that supports you and your students.

BENEFITS OF MIXED-SPEECH GROUPS

Now that I have squashed some negative beliefs you might be having about mixed groups, let's dive into more detail about the benefits of them. There are many benefits to mixed speech groups. Hopefully these points will help you view mixed groups differently:

- **Peer modeling:** Students benefit from observing and imitating peers who demonstrate stronger skills, providing natural examples of accurate speech, language use, or social interactions. Let your articulation students be language models. Let your language students be social skills models.
- **Increased opportunities for social skills practice:** Mixed groups simulate real-world communication contexts, allowing students to practice turn-taking, active listening, conversational exchanges, and perspective-taking in a supportive environment. Embrace the opportunities for discussion and working together. Do not fear too much chatter, we are SLPs after all!
- **Improved generalization:** Skills practiced in a group setting are more likely to transfer to other social environments, as students learn to use their skills in dynamic, multi-person interactions.
- **Time efficiency:** Working with multiple students at once allows SLPs to serve more students in less time while still addressing individual goals through group activities or rotations. With large caseloads, embrace this benefit. It will give you more time back.
- **Enhanced engagement:** Activities like games, discussions, competitions, or project-based learning can increase motivation and participation, as students often enjoy interacting with peers more than working alone. We are always looking for students to participate and be excited to come to speech. This is one way we can encourage that to happen.
- **Collaborative problem-solving:** Mixed groups encourage collaboration, with students learning to work together to solve problems, clarify instructions, or support one another, fostering a team dynamic.
- **Multifaceted learning opportunities:** Listening to different types of feedback (e.g., on articulation, language, or fluency) helps students build awareness of diverse communication strategies, even if they're not directly practicing that skill themselves.

- **Natural reinforcement and competition:** Group settings allow for positive peer reinforcement and friendly competition, motivating students to stay engaged and work toward their goals with enthusiasm.
- **Exposure to different communication styles:** Students in mixed groups learn to navigate and adapt to varied communication styles and needs, building flexibility and empathy in their interactions.
- **Dynamic and flexible therapy:** Mixed groups keep sessions lively and adaptable, challenging SLPs to think creatively while fostering a collaborative environment where each student can thrive.

By encouraging students to work together and learn from each other, they will build confidence since they will realize that other students struggle as well. Although students may have different language comprehension goals like summarizing or vocabulary, these skills are all necessary to be an effective and skilled reader and are practiced in the classroom as well. They can benefit from hearing others work on these goals. You might have a difficult time deciding what goals to work on when you have students who are deficient in so many skills. With mixed groups, they can be exposed to skills that aren't their goals and may even indirectly learn something.

The Process

This section explains a step-by-step process for working with mixed groups. Review the steps so you can see what areas you may need to improve on. The goal is to teach any group and feel confident that you can still make an impact.

Understand Student Goals and Group Dynamics

Review each student's IEP or individual goals before the session. Note overlapping skills (e.g., articulation and language) to plan activities that address multiple goals. Consider group dynamics such as personalities, abilities, and interaction styles to foster collaboration.

Plan Flexible, Goal-Driven Activities

Choose activities that can be adapted to different goals (e.g., a story or article for vocabulary, articulation, and sequencing). Build in layers of complexity, allowing students to engage at their individual levels while participating in the same task. Prepare visual supports, manipulatives, or scaffolding as needed.

Establish a Predictable Routine

Routines help students understand what to expect when they enter your speech room. How should they wait for their turn? What should they do if you are helping a peer? How should they behave if someone gets something wrong?

Some other routines you can use with a consistent structure to reduce anxiety and maximize focus:

- Warm-up: Quick activities targeting individual goals
- Group activity: Collaborative or parallel tasks addressing a range of goals
- Cool-down: Reinforcement or review to consolidate learning

Assign Clear Roles and Turn-Taking

Clearly define each student's role during the group activity (e.g., speaker, listener, question-asker). Use turn-taking strategies to ensure everyone has equal participation and time to practice their specific skills. Incorporate peer modeling, where students demonstrate for one another.

Use Multigoal Strategies

- Articulation: Have students practice target sounds within functional phrases or while responding to comprehension questions.
- Language: Embed vocabulary, syntax, or WH questions into activities (e.g., describing an image or retelling a story).
- Social skills: Focus on pragmatic language through group discussion, cooperative games, or role-playing.

Provide Individualized Feedback Within the Group

Give immediate, specific feedback tailored to each student's goal (e.g., correcting articulation for one while reinforcing turn-taking for another). Use private signals (e.g., thumbs-up or point cues) to discreetly support individual progress without disrupting the group.

Encourage Peer Interaction

Facilitate opportunities for students to learn from and support each other:

- Partner activities (e.g., asking/answering questions)
- Group problem-solving (e.g., working together on a puzzle or game)
- Praise and reinforce positive peer interactions.

Monitor and Document Progress

Use quick checklists, rubrics, or notes to track individual goal progress during each session.

Adjust and Differentiate in Real Time

Be flexible and prepared to adapt on the spot, such as increasing scaffolding for struggling students. Add challenges for those progressing quickly. Incorporate breaks or sensory supports as needed to maintain focus.

Reflect and Plan for Next Time

After the session, review what worked and what didn't. Modify future activities to better align with group dynamics or individual needs. Celebrate small wins and progress, both with students and yourself!

This process allows for efficient and meaningful therapy, balancing individual growth with the benefits of group interaction. Be flexible. Be willing to try new things. Be open to students working together.

SAMPLE LESSONS

This section includes two 30-minute sample lesson plans that you can use. One is with a YouTube video and the other is with an article, using any video or any article. I provided favorite resources for adapting plans in the previous chapter.

Lesson Plan: Using a YouTube Video to Enhance Communication Skills

Objective: Students will improve their articulation, language understanding, and social interaction skills.

Lesson Duration: 30 minutes

Materials:

- Selected YouTube video (Choose an engaging, content-appropriate video that includes dialogues, such as a scene from a popular educational series or documentary.)
- Projector or Smartboard for displaying the video
- Handouts with key vocabulary and phrases from the video
- Rubric for peer assessment

Step-by-Step Activities

1. **Introduction (3 minutes)**
   - Introduce the video topic, ensuring it aligns with students' interests and curricular goals.
   - Briefly outline the objectives for today's lesson, focusing on articulation, language comprehension, and social interactions.
2. **Watching the video (10 minutes)**
   - Play the selected YouTube video. Ensure subtitles are on to aid comprehension.
   - Pause briefly at key moments to highlight vocabulary and phrases important for the day's goals.
3. **Articulation and language activity (7 minutes)**
   - Have students repeat key sentences from the video to practice articulation.
   - Discuss the meaning of new vocabulary and phrases in context directly after repetition.
4. **Social skills mini role-play (7 minutes)**
   - Quickly organize students into pairs. Each pair chooses a short dialogue or interaction from the video to mimic.
   - Emphasize using clear speech and appropriate social interactions such as turn-taking.
5. **Discussion and closure (3 minutes)**
   - Conduct a brief class discussion on what they learned and observed.
   - Provide verbal feedback on articulation clarity, language use, and interaction quality.
   - Outline a follow-up activity or reflection to be completed at home, encouraging further engagement with the video content.

Assessment

- Informally assess articulation and language during the repetition and discussion activities.
- Observe social skills during the role-play, noting areas for improvement or commendation.

Adaptations for Different Needs

- For students needing more support, provide word banks or phrase lists during the articulation activity.
- Challenge advanced students by asking them to add sentences or use the vocabulary in new sentences.

Lesson Plan: Enhancing Communication Skills Through an Article

Objective: Students will improve their articulation, language understanding, and social interaction skills through reading and discussing an article.

Lesson Duration: 30 minutes

Materials:

- Selected article (choose an engaging and appropriate article that includes diverse vocabulary and is relevant to the students' curriculum or interests).
- Copies of the article for each student.
- Highlighters and pens.
- Discussion questions prepared in advance.
- Rubric for peer assessment.

Step-by-Step Activities

1. **Introduction (3 minutes)**
   - Introduce the topic of the article and its relevance to current curriculum or students' interests.
   - Outline the objectives for today's lesson, focusing on articulation, language comprehension, and social interactions.
2. **Reading the article (10 minutes)**
   - Distribute copies of the article. Have students read the article individually or in pairs.
   - Encourage them to highlight key vocabulary or sentences that they find interesting or challenging.
3. **Articulation and language discussion (7 minutes)**
   - Have students choose key sentences from the article to read aloud, focusing on clear articulation.
   - Discuss the meanings of highlighted vocabulary and any difficult phrases in context, asking students to paraphrase or use them in new sentences.
4. **Social skills through structured discussion (7 minutes)**
   - Break students into small groups and provide a set of discussion questions related to the article's content.
   - Instruct students to practice turn-taking and polite disagreement while discussing their thoughts on the article.

5. Closure and feedback (3 minutes)
- Bring the class back together and ask a few groups to share their discussion points.
- Provide verbal feedback on articulation, language use, and quality of interaction observed during the activities.
- Assign a brief reflective writing assignment for homework, asking students to summarize the article and reflect on their group discussion experience.

Assessment

- Conduct informal assessments during the reading aloud and discussion sessions to gauge articulation and comprehension.
- Observe social interactions during group discussions to assess social skills.

Adaptations for Different Needs

- Provide support such as glossaries or simplified versions of the article for students who need extra help.
- Encourage advanced students to explore deeper implications of the article or relate it to broader contexts.

DATA COLLECTION TIPS AND TRICKS

One question I get asked often is how to collect data with mixed groups. I went into detail about getting data in Chapter 5. However, it can be a challenge to collect data when you have mixed groups, so I share some tips and tricks related specifically to them. Remember, quality over quantity. This belief shift will make such an impact on the stress you put on data. Here are some tips for collecting data effectively in mixed groups, regardless of the group size:

- **Use a simple, organized data collection system:** Create a one-page tracking sheet with columns for each student's goals and include rows for tallying trials or noting observations.
  Use shorthand or symbols to save time (e.g., ✔ for correct, ✘ for incorrect, ↑ for progress). Prepare goal-specific templates in advance to minimize on-the-spot effort. I have provided some data collection forms on my resources page that you can access at www.speechtimefun.com/book.
- **Focus on one goal at a time per student:** While the group works on a shared activity, observe and collect data for one student's targeted goal during their turn. Rotate your focus among students, ensuring each has dedicated data

collection time without overwhelming yourself. I like to use a group data form and then transfer that over onto an individual data record sheet at the end of the day when I am reviewing the data and making my game plan for the next session. This group data form is available with the data forms on my resources page at www.speechtimefun.com/book.

- **Incorporate peer participation to extend data opportunities:** Assign one student as the "helper" to elicit responses from peers, allowing you to observe and document multiple interactions naturally. For example, if Student A asks a question, note Student B's response for language or articulation data while still engaging both. You will be surprised but students love to help collect data. The more they observe you doing it, the more they are aware what is going on. Especially with older students, they see you giving + and −. They know what is going on. Nothing to hide. Let them take turns helping you gather the data. They will feel empowered and find it fun.

- **Use technology for efficiency:** Use apps or digital tools to quickly tally data, record audio, or jot notes without disrupting the flow of the session. I have a digital data tool included with the SLP Elevate membership that allows you to enter data at the end of the session/day or even use a data logger and mark progress as it is happening.

- **Set data priorities for each session:** Predetermine which specific goals you'll focus on for each student during a session. This prevents you from trying to track everything at once. For example, focus on articulation trials for one student this session and language comprehension for another, while casually noting progress on other goals. Remember, you cannot work on all the goals a student has in one session.

These tips allow you to efficiently balance data collection with active engagement, ensuring meaningful progress tracking in a mixed group setting. Remember, the more specific the goal, the easier it is to measure, especially in a mixed group. The more you understand how to work on that goal, the more progress you will measure, even with fewer trials. Remember, one trial is still data. Especially with comprehension goals, where you are reading one article most of the session, you may only have one opportunity to demonstrate progress in a session, and that is sufficient.

HAVING FUN WITH MIXED GROUPS

Mixed groups aren't something to fear, they are something to embrace. When you approach mixed speech groups with curiosity and confidence, you'll see how powerful they can be. Students stay engaged, they learn from each other, and planning becomes more efficient. In fact, I often find that group sessions are faster-paced and require less preparation than individual ones. Plus, students love the opportunity to interact with their peers. They would rather talk to each other than to me, and I am totally okay with that! Group sessions create a natural space for connection, communication, and collaboration. When students are talking, laughing, and learning together, they don't feel so alone in their struggles. They are reminded that learning can be fun. Even if progress takes time, they are showing up, participating, and building confidence. That is always a win for me in any session.

NOW WHAT?

It is time to self-reflect on your views on mixed groups and think about how you have been approaching them so far. Take a second to answer some of these thought-provoking questions:

- How did you feel about mixed groups before reading this chapter?
- What can you let go of so you can view mixed groups differently?
- What will you try so you can see how mixed groups can be beneficial?
- What has been your biggest obstacle in embracing mixed groups?
- How might peer interactions in your groups benefit students more than individual work?
- What is one belief about mixed groups you're ready to let go of?

Time to take action!

- Test one of the sample lesson plans in your next session and jot down what worked and what didn't.
- Choose a single versatile piece of material and brainstorm three different ways to use it in your next mixed group.
- Try a new data collection method.

You won't know unless you try. See how students respond. Put some reminders on a sticky note: connection over data collection; one trial is still data; if I have fun they will too; and mixed groups are fun. Remember, mixed groups aren't a problem to solve—they're an opportunity to innovate, connect, and create a unique rhythm in your therapy sessions. Embrace the challenge and watch your students—and yourself—thrive!

CHAPTER 13

Building Articulation and Social Skills

For most of this book, I have focused heavily on language comprehension goals. I did this for many reasons. It is an area that most SLPs are not comfortable with, most secondary students are working on these goals, and it is an area I feel most comfortable with. Most of my secondary students had those goals themselves. I used the strategies in this book to work with them, get them quick wins, and see tons of progress. This chapter discusses other common goal areas and ways you can address them in motivating and easy-to-prepare ways.

ARTICULATION IDEAS FOR SECONDARY STUDENTS

By the time students reach middle or high school, working on articulation goals can feel. . .complicated. As SLPs, we often find ourselves supporting students who have been working on the same sounds for years, maybe even since early elementary school. It is no surprise that by this age, they are tired of it. They are aware of it. And in many cases, they are over it!

You might hear things like "I don't even care anymore," or "Why am I still doing this?" Honestly, it is a fair question. These students have grown up, matured, and moved into classrooms where social pressure is real. They want to blend in with their peers. They want to talk about things that are relevant to them, not just repeat /r/ words 10 times in a row. And yet, here they are, still needing support with a sound that won't stick. Oftentimes, they are forced to continue with speech due to a parent's concern, but it isn't something they are motivated by or want to address themselves.

At this stage, SLPs are rarely drilling isolated sounds or single words. Instead, they are focusing on helping students use their target sounds correctly in sentences and conversation. They're looking at generalization and carry-over—those final, often stubborn steps of articulation therapy. They are helping students notice when they are not using their sound and learn how to correct themselves in real time. In short, they are building self-awareness, self-monitoring, and self-correction skills. These skills will give students ownership and independence.

This chapter is designed to help you make articulation work feel different for your older students. The goal isn't just to make progress, but to make it meaningful and relevant. The activities you will find here are designed with age-respectful themes, real-word application, and a whole lot of intention behind how you support your students. When a student has been on this journey for years, they don't just need more practice. They need to feel like their efforts matter and that they are finally getting closer to the finish line.

The goal is for your lessons to be fun, relevant, and related to your students' worlds. I once asked a sixth grader to practice articulation drills, and they stared at me like I'd suggested we recite Shakespeare together. That's when I realized I needed to bring in TikTok scripts and song lyrics to get their attention. You should encourage your students to self-reflect and self-monitor at this age.

Here are some ideas you can use to work on any sound, in any position, and which can be used at any level. You can pair these ideas with minimal pairs, auditory bombardment, visual cues, and other strategies.

- **Articulation joke books:** Have students look up free jokes for kids on the internet. Have them find ones bombarded with their speech sounds. They can create a joke book with paper, printed on a computer, or even just using a file folder. They can practice telling jokes with their group.
- **100 trial races:** We are always trying to get high trials with our articulation students. You can use dice (even the high-numbered dice) to get high trials. Students can mark off their trials until they get to 100. You can use graph paper to mark it off, a hole puncher and get 100 holes, or even mark it off with candy. Who can get to 100 first?
- **Articulation word searches:** Who doesn't love a word search? You can make them easily online using a free word search creator at https://puzzlemaker .discoveryeducation.com/word-search. You can even have students make one themselves. Create lists with their target words, generate a word search, and see who can find the words the fastest.
- **Articulation Mad Libs:** Mad Libs are a great way to practice vocabulary and parts of speech, but they can also be used to work on articulation. Have students fill in all their words using words with their sound. You can prepare by generating parts of speech lists with their sounds to use as a word bank. They can practice their sounds as they are selecting them and again when they are

reading their finished projects. You can find free Mad Libs games online at https://kids.nationalgeographic.com/games/funny-fill-in.

- **Pop culture articulation debates:** If your students love pop culture, use it to motivate them and encourage them to practice their articulation targets. First, choose popular topics like favorite music artists, video games, movies, or social media trends. Then, students can pick a side in a debate (e.g., "Which is the best streaming platform?"). They can practice their articulation targets while making their points and rebuttals.
- **Podcast or TikTok script practice:** With this activity, students can practice their sounds with a format that is familiar, enjoyable, and relatable. Have students write and perform a short script for a fictional podcast or TikTok, focusing on a topic they love (e.g., sports, fashion, memes). Students can perform their script while practicing their articulation targets. You can even let them use simple props or record their work for a class "podcast showcase" or mock social media post critique. This is a great way to self-reflect on their production of their target sounds.
- **Movie voiceover challenge:** Do you have the next movie voiceover star in your therapy room? Have students that love to recite lines from popular movies? Use it to your advantage. Have a contest for the best movie voiceover and mimic the lines of their favorite movies. Choose popular movie scenes or trailers with clear dialogue and bombarded with their articulation target sounds (e.g., superhero speeches, dramatic monologues). Students can practice delivering the lines. You can even compare their lines and versions to the originals. Who said it best?
- **Lyrics articulation showdown:** Students can practice their articulation targets while reciting their favorite song lyrics. Pick clean and popular song lyrics with quick or challenging diction (e.g., rap verses, pop hits). Students can take turns reciting the lyrics, focusing on clear articulation rather than singing. For a competitive twist, have a speed round to see who can articulate the lyrics most clearly at a faster pace. You can even end the session with a karaoke session and play the song's sing-along version on YouTube. You can find so many song lyrics free online.
- **Social media influencer simulation:** Students are often motivated by social media and influencers, so why not use these tools? It is a relatable context for them. Have students create a short, 30-second "influencer pitch" for a product or cause they care about. They can practice their articulation and use enthusiasm as if they were speaking to an audience online.
- **Gaming commentary practice:** This is another relatable context for them. Choose a popular video game (or a related topic, like esports) and have students

act as live commentators. They can describe gameplay, strategies, or their favorite aspects of the game as if they're hosting a stream or competition. You can even pair students so one acts as the gamer while the other narrates, then switch roles.

DIVING DEEPER INTO THE SOCIAL MEDIA INFLUENCER SIMULATION

For most students, this is an engaging activity. This section discusses some examples to help you visualize these activities with your students.

Sample Scripts for a Social Media Influencer Simulation

Sample Script: "Reusable Water Bottle Campaign" for /r/

Introduction (initial /r/): "Hey everyone! I'm here to talk about an awesome way to stay hydrated and help the Earth at the same time! Meet the *Reusable Rainforest Bottle!* It's the perfect choice for reducing waste and staying refreshed wherever you go."

Features and benefits (medial /r/): "This bottle is durable, portable, and keeps your drinks super cold. Plus, for every bottle you buy, a tree gets planted in the rainforest. Pretty cool, right?"

Call to action (final /r/): "So, whether you're at the park, the library, or the gym, grab your *Reusable Rainforest Bottle* today! Click the link below to order now!"

Sample Script: "Chocolate Chip Energy Bars" for /ch/

Introduction (initial /ch/): "Hey, friends! Are you always on the go but need a quick and cheerful snack to fuel your day? Let me introduce you to the best snack ever—Chocolate Chip Crunch Bars!"

Features and benefits (Medial /ch/): "These bars are packed with protein, oats, and, of course, rich chocolate chips. They're perfect for munching between classes, at practice, or while you're chilling with friends."

Call to action (Final /ch/): "So don't wait! Catch your own box of Chocolate Chip Crunch Bars today and crunch your way to better energy. Click the link below to purchase now!"

Sample Script: "Super Shine Shampoo" for /sh/

Introduction (initial /sh/): "Hey, everyone! Are you tired of dull, lifeless hair? I've got something special for you—introducing *Super Shine Shampoo!* This is the shampoo that will make your hair *shine* like never before!"

Features and benefits (medial /sh/): "Super Shine Shampoo is packed with nourishing oils and vitamins that leave your hair soft, silky, and *shimmering*. And the best part? It smells like a tropical *paradise*. One *wash* and you'll be hooked!"

Call to action (final /sh/): "Don't let dull hair steal your spotlight! Grab your bottle of *Super Shine Shampoo* now, and give your hair the love it deserves. Swipe up to purchase!"

Sample Script: "Lemon Luxe Lotion" for /l/

Introduction (initial /l/): "Hello, lovely friends! Are you looking for a lotion that keeps your skin feeling fresh and fabulous? Let me introduce you to *Lemon Luxe Lotion*! It's lightweight, luxurious, and loaded with natural lemon extracts!"

Features and benefits (medial /l/): "Lemon Luxe Lotion is silky smooth and absorbs like a dream! Say goodbye to dry, flaky skin and hello to a glow that lasts all day long. Plus, the light lemon scent leaves you feeling calm and collected."

Call to action (final /l/): "Don't let dry skin hold you back! Grab your bottle of *Lemon Luxe Lotion* today and level up your skincare game. Swipe up to shop now!"

Instructions for students:

1. **Draft their script:** Have them brainstorm a product, real or fictional, that they care about or find interesting.
2. **Highlight words:** Help them identify their sounds in initial, medial, and final positions to target in their pitch.
3. **Practice:** Guide them through practicing their script with feedback on their articulation target (e.g., tongue position, vocal clarity).
4. **Perform and reflect:** Record their performance, play it back, and encourage them to self-monitor their production.

Reflection questions post-activity:

- How did it feel to focus on your sounds during your pitch?
- Were there any words that were more challenging?
- What strategies helped you the most to produce your sound?
- How could you use what you learned today in real-life conversations?

Sample Script for Gaming Commentary Targeting /r/

Racing Royale

Introduction (initial /r/): "Welcome, racers! We're live at the ultimate *Racing Royale*! Get ready to rev those engines and race through rugged roads, rapid rivers, and risky ramps."

Gameplay description (medial /r/): "Right now, Ryan's racing a red car, and it's roaring past the competition! He just cleared a crazy curve with incredible control. Up ahead, there's a dangerous bridge with broken railings. Will he make it? Oh no, he nearly crashed!"

Exciting finish (final /r/): "And here we are at the final corner! The racers are neck-and-neck, giving their all. Ryan roars ahead at the last second—what a victory! What an unforgettable *Racing Royale*!"

Sample Script for Gaming Commentary Targeting /s/

A Fast-Paced Racing Game

"Speeding down the straightaway, the shiny silver car is in second place! Watch as it swiftly slides around the sharp turn. Oh no! It's about to hit a sand trap! The driver slams the brakes just in time and saves the race!"

"Now, heading toward the finish line, the car is spinning through a tricky section. Can it stay on the smooth track? The suspense is so intense you can feel the sizzle in the air!"

"There's the flag! The driver scores a stunning second place victory! That was a spectacular race, full of slick strategies and smart maneuvers!"

Suggestions for Teaching and Using Gaming Commentary with Any Articulation Sound

Preparation:

- **Word bank:** Create a list of target words with the sound in various positions (e.g., initial, medial, final). Tailor words to gaming themes (e.g., /r/: *race, run, restart*).
- **Model the sound:** Demonstrate proper articulation and practice in isolation using tools like mirrors or tactile feedback.

Practice:

- **Warm-up:** Start with target words in isolation, then move to short phrases or sentences (e.g., /sh/: "The ship is rushing through the waves!").
- **Scaffold complexity:** Gradually increase from words to full sentences and spontaneous commentary.

Activity implementation:

- **Choose a game:** Use live games, recorded gameplay, or made-up scenarios that fit student interests.
- **Commentary practice:** Students narrate gameplay, using as many target words as possible, focusing on articulation and expression.
- **Role-playing:** Pair students as "gamer" and "commentator" to practice target sounds collaboratively.

Feedback and reflection:

- **Record and review:** Record commentary for self-assessment and feedback, focusing on clear articulation.
- **Peer feedback:** Encourage students to give constructive feedback to each other.

Follow-up:

- **Increase challenge:** Add timers, more complex vocabulary, or spontaneous commentary to simulate live scenarios.
- **Creative extensions:** Let students design their own game or script commentary with target sounds.
- **Incorporate literacy:** Include reading or writing scripts to reinforce sound practice in written language.

SOCIAL SKILLS IDEAS FOR SECONDARY STUDENTS

It's important to ensure that your secondary students are motivated by the social skill goals you set and that they are appropriate for this age group. This isn't a book on neurodiversity-affirming practices or social skills goal-writing, but you do need to make sure you are not pushing students to do anything that is uncomfortable or inappropriate. These goals and activities should have your students' best interests at heart. The social skills activities I share here can be used to work on any goal.

Using Commercials

I love using commercials to work on comprehension skills like inferencing. But I also love using them for social skills. They are short, funny, and relatable. This is where we teach students to decode messages and realize why they *really* want that $8 latte.

- You can work on nonverbal communication by analyzing body language, facial expressions, tone of voice, and gestures used by actors. Pause a commercial at key moments and ask students to interpret the emotions or intentions of the characters based on nonverbal cues.
- You can work on perspective taking. Consider how characters in the commercial might feel or think, and why. Discuss why a character or spokesperson might behave a certain way and how their actions aim to connect with the audience.
- You can work on recognizing persuasive techniques and strategies used to influence opinions (e.g., appeal to emotions, authority, or trends). Identify persuasive elements in commercials and discuss how they might affect different audiences. This can tie into understanding how messages are received based on individual perspectives.
- You can work on working as a team. Students can work together to interpret or critique a commercial. Students can analyze a commercial and present their findings on its social message, target audience, and persuasive techniques.

Using Games

- You can work on communication skills such as clear expression of ideas, active listening, asking clarifying questions using games such as Charades, Pictionary, or collaborative storytelling games. Encourage students to explain their ideas effectively and listen to others to achieve common goals.
- You can work on teamwork and collaboration by having students working together, dividing roles, supporting teammates, and resolving conflicts. You can use games like escape rooms to have students working together for a common goal.
- You can work on emotional regulation such as managing frustration, handling competition, and staying calm under pressure using competitive games like Uno!, Jenga, or fast-paced card games. Teach coping strategies for losing, dealing with setbacks, and showing good sportsmanship.
- You can work on nonverbal communication such as reading body language, facial expressions, and gestures using Charades, Heads Up!, or silent strategy games. Improve awareness of nonverbal cues and how they influence interactions.

- You can work on building empathy and understanding others' feelings and experiences. using story-driven video games, role-playing games, or empathy card games like The Ungame. Use gameplay to explore emotions and practice empathizing with characters or teammates.

Using Real Photos

You can find images described below with Google Images:

- You can work on interpreting nonverbal cues like body language, facial expressions, and posture. Show photos of people in different scenarios (e.g., a person smiling, someone looking stressed) and ask students to interpret how the individuals might be feeling based on nonverbal cues.
- You can work on perspective taking by understanding the emotions, motivations, and experiences of others. Present a photo and ask students to create a short story about what might have happened before or after the moment captured, focusing on the perspectives of the individuals in the photo.
- You can work on conversational skills by generating questions or comments to engage with others. Provide a photo and ask students to practice starting a conversation based on what they observe. (e.g., "That looks like a fun event—have you ever been to something similar?")
- You can work on cultural awareness by appreciating and understanding diversity in social interactions. Use photos from different cultural events or traditions and discuss what students can learn about communication, norms, or values from those images.
- You can work on understanding group dynamics such as recognizing roles, relationships, and interactions within a group. Show a photo of a team or group working together and have students identify who might be leading, who seems engaged, and who might need support.

These are just various activities that you can use to work on a variety of social skills goals. You can easily adapt some skills from one activity and apply them to another. These activities are built for secondary students, and they will see how they can use these skills outside your therapy room walls.

PUTTING IT ALL TOGETHER

Articulation and social skills activities don't have to be fancy or elaborate. They just need to be relevant to students' worlds. Most of the activities described in this chapter only require Google Images, lyrics from the internet, YouTube videos, or simple props. They take minutes to prepare. By learning your students' interests and personal goals, you can easily decide which activities to utilize. If you want them to be motivated, you need them to understand the relevance of what they're learning.

NOW WHAT?

Take the time to reflect on these questions:

- Which activity resonates most with your students' interests?
- How can you involve students in choosing the themes or materials for their sessions?
- What's one new activity you're excited to try, and how will you adapt it for your students' specific goals?

Try one of the activities for articulation or social skills. Pick one that relates to the interests and personal goals of your students. You may be surprised to learn more about your students and their desires, goals, and dreams. You may be surprised to see how easy it is to plan a motivating session that gets laughs, participating, and progress.

Remember, progress is a journey, not a sprint. As you incorporate these creative activities into your sessions, remember that every small win is a win. Whether it's a clearer sound, a burst of confidence, or an excited student, it is a step toward your students' success. You're not just teaching articulation; you're helping your students find their voice and feel empowered to use it in the real world. That is the key difference between working with older students and younger students.

Be patient with yourself and your students. Some days will be easier than others, but every effort counts. Celebrate the moments of laughter, the sparks of understanding, and the courage your students show when they try something new. You're making a difference, one sound at a time. Keep going—you've got this!

CHAPTER 14

What About Life Skills?

This book would not be complete without discussing life skills. As SLPs, we get to support these students' language and communication skills in a way that is relevant and beneficial for them. We get to support them as they are building their independence. Functional communication and independence is essential for this population.

WHY FUNCTIONAL COMMUNICATION AND INDEPENDENCE?

Functional communication and independence is what successful intervention for middle and high school life skills students is all about. These areas represent the practical, real-world applications of language and communication, focusing on empowering students to navigate daily life with confidence and autonomy. This section explains why these areas are essential.

Functional Communication: Building Bridges to the World

Functional communication refers to the ability to express needs, wants, thoughts, and emotions effectively in real-world situations. For life skills students, this goes beyond academic or rote language skills—it's about making meaningful connections with others and navigating their environment.

- **Meeting basic needs:** Functional communication enables students to express hunger, discomfort, preferences, or the need for assistance. Whether through verbal speech, AAC devices, or gestures, this skill ensures that students' most basic needs are met without frustration or miscommunication.
- **Fostering relationships:** Being able to greet peers, engage in small talk, or participate in shared activities helps students build friendships and feel included

in social environments. Communication is the gateway to forming connections and reducing isolation.

- **Advocating for themselves:** Teaching students to ask for help, clarify instructions, or negotiate a solution in a conflict fosters self-advocacy. This skill is crucial for their safety, well-being, and success in diverse settings like the classroom, workplace, or community.

- **Participating in the community:** Functional communication empowers students to order food at a restaurant, ask for directions, or handle transactions. These small acts contribute to a sense of belonging and independence in the community.

Independence: The Ultimate Goal

Independence isn't about achieving perfection—it's about empowering students to make decisions, solve problems, and take ownership of their lives to the best of their abilities. Independence reinforces their confidence, reduces reliance on caregivers, and opens up opportunities for success.

- **Decision-making:** Independence starts with choices. Teaching students to make decisions—what to eat, what to wear, and how to spend their time—helps them feel empowered and in control of their lives.

- **Navigating the real world:** Skills like reading bus schedules, following a recipe, and managing a budget are critical for students to thrive beyond school. These are the building blocks of adult life and give students the tools to participate fully in their communities.

- **Employment readiness:** Independence in communication and tasks prepares students for the workplace. From understanding instructions to interacting with coworkers, these skills are vital for securing and maintaining a job.

- **Confidence and self-worth:** Every step toward independence, no matter how small, reinforces a student's sense of self-worth. They begin to see themselves as capable individuals who can contribute meaningfully to their environments.

The SLP's Role

As SLPs, we have the unique opportunity to blend communication skills with functional tasks that directly impact students' lives. We don't just teach words; we teach how to use them in meaningful ways. We don't just model actions; we build pathways for independence.

- **Real-world focus:** Therapy goals should prioritize skills that students will use daily—whether it's asking for a bathroom break, initiating a conversation, or following a recipe.
- **Holistic support:** Collaborate with families, teachers, and job coaches to ensure that students are practicing these skills in multiple settings. Consistency across environments accelerates mastery.
- **Empowerment through communication:** When students can express themselves and participate in their world, they gain confidence and a sense of control. This empowerment transforms not just their communication but their entire outlook on life.

Functional communication and independence are not just therapy objectives; they are life objectives. By focusing on these areas, we prepare students for a fulfilling and autonomous life. This approach celebrates their strengths, addresses their challenges and builds a foundation for lifelong growth and participation in the world around them.

UNDERSTANDING STUDENTS' UNIQUE CHALLENGES

Working with middle and high school life skills students presents a distinct set of challenges, ranging from communication barriers to social stigmas, and varying levels of cognitive and physical abilities. Recognizing these challenges and developing strategies to address them is key to supporting these students effectively. This section discusses some common challenges and actionable steps you can take to overcome them.

Diverse Communication Needs

Life skills students often have a wide range of communication abilities, from nonverbal to verbal communicators, and they may rely on various tools like AAC devices, gestures, or visual supports. This diversity requires individualized approaches to meet their needs.

What SLPs can do:

- **Conduct thorough assessments:** Evaluate each student's strengths, challenges, and preferred communication methods. Use dynamic assessments to understand their functional communication in real-world scenarios.

- **Use multimodal communication:** Incorporate a mix of AAC, visual supports, and verbal communication strategies to provide students with multiple ways to express themselves.
- **Focus on functional goals:** Instead of targeting isolated language skills, prioritize functional communication goals that directly impact daily life, such as requesting help, making choices, or navigating social interactions.

Social Stigma and Confidence Issues

Many life skills students face social stigma from peers, which can lead to low self-esteem and reluctance to participate in social activities or communication tasks.

What SLPs can do:

- **Build a safe environment:** Create a therapy space where students feel respected, valued, and celebrated for their progress. Emphasize a strengths-based approach to build confidence.
- **Incorporate peer models:** Pair life skills students with supportive peers who can model appropriate social behavior and foster inclusion.
- **Practice real-world scenarios:** Role-play common social interactions (e.g., introducing themselves, ordering at a restaurant) to help students build confidence in practical communication settings.

Limited Generalization of Skills

Students often struggle to apply skills learned in therapy to other settings, such as the classroom, home, or community.

What SLPs can do:

- **Integrate therapy across environments:** Collaborate with teachers, paraprofessionals, and families to ensure consistent use of communication strategies across all settings.
- **Teach in context:** Incorporate real-life activities into therapy, such as practicing money exchanges, following directions in a kitchen setting, or using public transportation.
- **Use visual schedules and prompts:** Help students understand when and how to use their skills by providing visual supports that outline expectations for various environments.

Varied Cognitive Abilities

Life skills students often have a wide range of cognitive abilities, which can make it difficult to design lessons that are both accessible and appropriately challenging.

What SLPs can do:

- **Differentiate instruction:** Adapt materials and instructions to match each student's cognitive level, using concrete examples, simplified language, or scaffolding as needed. You don't need to start from scratch and reinvent the wheel for every student. This is modifying what you have so you can use it and move forward. You can build in scaffolding like sentence starters, choices, or visual aids to give them an opportunity to be successful with the materials presented. Keep the heart of the activity, but change the way they can access it.
- **Focus on strengths:** Build on what students already know and enjoy engaging them in new learning opportunities. For example, if a student loves cooking, integrate recipes into therapy sessions.
- **Break tasks into steps:** Use task analysis to break down complex skills into smaller, manageable steps. This approach helps students feel successful at each stage of the process.

Behavioral Challenges

Students may exhibit behaviors like refusal, distraction, or frustration, often stemming from communication difficulties or sensory sensitivities.

What SLPs can do:

- **Understand the behavior's function:** Determine if the behavior is a form of communication, a response to sensory overload, or a sign of frustration. Address the underlying cause rather than just the behavior.
- **Provide clear expectations:** Use visual schedules, first-then boards, or social stories to help students understand what is expected of them during therapy.
- **Reinforce positive behavior:** Use positive reinforcement to encourage participation, such as praise, tokens, or preferred activities.

Balancing Academic and Functional Goals

There is often pressure coming from administration, parents, or colleagues to address academic skills, even when students' primary needs lie in functional communication and life skills.

What SLPs can do:

- **Advocate for functional priorities:** Work with IEP teams to emphasize goals that will have the greatest impact on students' daily lives, such as ordering food, participating in conversations, or following a routine.
- **Blend academic and functional goals:** Incorporate academic concepts into functional tasks. For example, teach counting skills through money exchanges or literacy skills through reading recipes.
- **Educate stakeholders:** Share data and examples of how functional communication directly supports academic engagement and independence.

Limited Resources

Schools often lack specialized materials, tools, or training for working with life skills students, which can make therapy planning and implementation more difficult.

What SLPs can do:

- **Leverage free or low-cost resources:** Use community resources, free online materials, or everyday items (e.g., grocery store flyers, bus schedules) as therapy tools.
- **Collaborate with staff and families:** Partner with teachers, job coaches, and families to share resources and ideas for reinforcing skills across environments.
- **Invest in professional development:** Attend workshops, webinars, or conferences focused on working with life skills students to stay informed about evidence-based practices.

Transitioning to Adulthood

Life skills students face unique challenges as they prepare to transition from school to adult life, such as finding employment, managing daily living tasks, and accessing community services.

What SLPs can do:

- **Incorporate vocational training:** Practice job-related communication skills, such as interviewing, following instructions, or engaging with coworkers, in therapy sessions.
- **Teach self-advocacy:** Help students learn to express their needs, preferences, and boundaries in different settings, from the workplace to medical appointments.

■ **Connect with community resources:** Collaborate with transition coordinators, job coaches, and local organizations to ensure students have access to postsecondary support.

By addressing these challenges with thoughtful strategies and a collaborative mindset, SLPs can help life skills students achieve meaningful progress, fostering their ability to communicate effectively, build relationships, and navigate the world with greater independence.

WHAT ABOUT AAC USERS?

When working with students who use AAC, one of the most important things to remember is that you can use materials that you are already using with your other life skills students. With a few thoughtful adaptations, you can use the same materials and spend less time preparing.

AAC users often have similar goals as their peers, such as building vocabulary, increasing communication functions (beyond requesting), and developing social interaction skills. The difference is in how they access and express language. Rather than creating something entirely new, focus on adapting what you already have to support these goals with their communication style.

Here are a few simple ways you can adapt your existing materials for AAC users:

1. Preprogram target vocabulary into their device or prepare a low-tech board with keywords for the activity. For example, if you are doing a cooking activity, make sure you provide vocabulary such as "mix," "pour," and "bowl" so that the student can participate and comment throughout the activity.
2. Model language throughout the activity using their AAC system. If the class is discussing community helpers, model phrases such as "I see a firefighter" as you point to the relevant symbols. Try to use your own device and not theirs and avoid hand-over hand modeling, since it may feel invasive and not neurodiversity affirming.
3. Give visual and motor-friendly response options. Instead of asking open-ended questions that require verbal responses, offer AAC-accessible choices such as "Do you want to watch or help?"

You are still working toward meaningful communication goals, just supporting access in a way that makes participation possible. If you are looking for ready-to-use

AAC materials or visuals to adapt your current activities, here are a few great (and free) resources worth checking out:

- www.aaclanguagelab.com: This website is great for language goals and includes free lesson plans and activities based on AAC language stages.
- www.project-core.com: This site offers free universal core boards, implementation strategies, and printable materials for use.
- www.saltillo.com/chatcorner: You can access free downloadable activities, books, and communication boards that align with common classroom themes.

With a few small adjustments and the right supports, your AAC users can be fully included in meaningful, engaging activities right alongside their peers.

INCORPORATING VOCATIONAL THEMES

Working with themes can make therapy planning easier, more relevant, and fun for the students. Using vocational themes allows your therapy to integrate to the curriculum of the life skills classroom. You provide your students with language and communication skills that are necessary for life outside of school. Consider these themes that you can incorporate and use with your life skills students:

- **Teaching workplace communication skills:** You can work on greeting coworkers, asking for help, and understanding instructions. You can also practice appropriate tone, volume, and body language.
- **Simulating real-world scenarios:** This can include role-play tasks such as taking food orders, stocking shelves, or sorting mail. You can use scripts, visual aids, or AAC devices for scaffolding.
- **Collaborating with community partners:** You can partner with local businesses for job-shadowing or volunteer opportunities. Incorporate feedback from job coaches or employers into therapy goals.

Practical Therapy Ideas

I am all about practical therapy ideas that are easy to prep and relevant to students. Here are some ideas you can easily use to target a variety of speech and language goals.

Cooking

Cooking involves more than just putting ingredients together to make a meal! Students also need to learn to shop, meal plan, and follow directions to make a recipe. Here are a few fun activities that students can do during speech time:

- Look for recipes that they would like to make using cookbooks or the internet.
- Use sales circulars or online shopping apps to pick out the ingredients they will need.
- Put the cut-out steps to the recipe in the proper order by sequencing them.

Reading Medication Information

When students are working toward living independently, they need to learn to take medication correctly. Here are some activities they can do to plan out how much medication to take and when:

- Read the directions on the medication packaging. These can be printed out so that the student can highlight the time and dosage on them.
- Match dosage amounts. Students can fill medicine cups with water to match the amount of medication listed on the packaging.
- Use a clock to figure out what time to take the medication. For example, if the packaging says, "every 12 hours," then the student can figure out what time to take the medication again if they took it at 8:00 am.

Reading and Ordering from a Menu

This task is especially important if the student has any food allergies! Menus can be printed off restaurant websites for these activities:

- Have the student complete a menu scavenger hunt! Most menus have categories in similar locations. Students can locate where the drinks are listed, where the appetizers are located, and so on.
- Work on using pictures to find items. For example, soft drink logos will often be found on a menu where the drinks are listed. These can help the student find things that they want.
- Work on locating headings on menus.
- Practice conversations with a server. Have your student identify what they want from the menu and practice ordering while you role-play a server.

Taking Public Transportation

Another part of vocational training is accessing public transportation. However, bus and rail schedules can be confusing! Here's how to work on them with students:

- Use a map to identify what route the student needs to take. Most routes are color-coded, which makes it easier.
- Identify the student's stop. This is a good opportunity to review the student's address with them.
- Using a highlighter, work with the student to highlight the timetable that the student will need to use.
- Practice with the student and then take away some of the scaffolding by giving the student other routes to plan out.

Interviewing

Interviewing is a big part of vocational training! Here are some interview skills to work on during speech time.

- Practice nonverbal communication such as posture, eye contact, and tone.
- Identify the student's skills and abilities.
- Ask questions about work times, salary, and work responsibilities.
- Ask questions to clarify information.
- Memorize personal information, such as the student's address and phone number (for the company's paperwork).

Collaboration with Families

Families are essential partners in supporting the progress and independence of life skills students. By involving families in goal setting, data tracking, and ensuring carry-over across settings, SLPs can create a more cohesive and impactful therapy experience. This section includes ways to strengthen collaboration with families and maximize student success.

Inviting Family Input for Goal-Setting

Why it's important: Families have unique insights into their child's abilities, challenges, and daily routines. Their input ensures that therapy goals are relevant, functional, and aligned with the student's home and community environments.

Strategies for collaboration:

- **Start with conversations:** Schedule regular check-ins (e.g., phone calls, meetings, or surveys) to discuss family priorities, concerns, and observations. Example questions to ask families:
  - What communication skills are most important for your child at home?
  - Are there specific tasks or settings where you feel additional support is needed?
  - What would independence look like for your child in your family's daily life?
- **Include families in the IEP process:** Encourage families to actively participate in IEP meetings by sharing their perspective on goals and identifying areas they feel are crucial for long-term success.
- **Use a strengths-based approach:** Highlight the student's abilities when discussing goals, showing how therapy can build on these strengths to address challenges. For instance, if a student enjoys cooking at home, a goal might focus on requesting ingredients or following verbal instructions in a kitchen setting.

Collaborating on Data Tracking

Families can provide valuable information about how a student uses communication skills outside of therapy, offering insights into generalization and progress.

Strategies for collaboration:

- **Develop a simple data-sharing system:** Create a shared communication log, Google Form, or app where families can record observations or rate skills in real-life contexts. Keep it simple and user-friendly to encourage consistent use. Example: A parent might log whether their child independently requested an item or used a new AAC symbol at home.
- **Share progress regularly:** Provide families with clear, jargon-free updates about their child's progress, highlighting both successes and areas of focus. Example: "This week, Jamie successfully used their AAC device to greet peers during a group activity. We're now working on expanding this skill to ask for help."
- **Provide checklists:** Offer families short, specific checklists or prompts to track targeted skills during daily routines, such as:
  - Did your child ask for help when needed?
  - Did they use full sentences when ordering at a restaurant?

Ensuring Carry-over Across Settings

For therapy to be truly effective, students need to generalize communication skills to real-world environments, including home, school, and the community.

Strategies for collaboration:

- **Provide home practice activities:** Share practical, easy-to-implement activities that align with therapy goals and fit into the family's routines. Example: "While grocery shopping, encourage your child to ask where items are located or check off items on the list using their AAC device."
- **Create visual supports for home use:** Provide families with visual aids, such as communication boards, schedules, or social stories, to reinforce therapy strategies at home. Example: A visual checklist for getting ready in the morning could include steps like brushing teeth, packing a lunch, and putting on shoes, with opportunities to practice requesting help or commenting.
- **Model strategies for families:** Demonstrate how to use specific techniques, such as prompting or reinforcement, so families feel confident in supporting communication at home. Example: Show a parent how to pause after asking a question to give their child more processing time before responding.
- **Encourage role-playing at home:** Suggest scenarios that families can practice, such as ordering food, asking for directions, or participating in family conversations.

Building a Two-Way Partnership

Collaboration works best when families and SLPs see each other as equal partners, each contributing unique expertise to the student's success.

Strategies for collaboration:

- **Create a judgment-free zone:** Acknowledge that families may have limited time or resources and work with them to find practical, realistic solutions.
- **Offer flexibility:** Adapt communication methods to meet the family's needs, whether through email updates, video demonstrations, or quick check-ins during pick-up/drop-off.
- **Celebrate wins together:** Share even small victories with families, reinforcing their role in their child's progress and building trust. Example: "Sam confidently ordered their own drink at lunch today! I know you've been practicing this at home—it really shows!"

Empowering Families as Advocates

Families are often the most consistent advocates for their child. By equipping them with knowledge and tools, SLPs can empower families to support their child's needs across settings.

Strategies for collaboration:

- **Educate about communication rights:** Teach families about their child's right to communication support in all environments, including school, extra-curriculars, and community settings.
- **Provide advocacy tools:** Share scripts or templates for families to use when advocating for accommodations or support, such as requesting AAC training for staff or ensuring communication-friendly environments.
- **Involve families in strategy selection:** Encourage families to share feedback on what strategies work best at home, fostering a sense of ownership in their child's progress.

Collaborating with families is a cornerstone of success for life skills students. By involving families in goal-setting, data tracking, and carry-over strategies, you can create a unified approach that empowers students to thrive in all areas of life. When families feel heard, supported, and equipped with tools to reinforce progress, the impact extends far beyond the therapy room.

FINDING APPROPRIATE RESOURCES FOR MIDDLE AND HIGH SCHOOL LIFE SKILLS STUDENTS

Working with middle and high school life skills students often requires age-appropriate and functional resources that align with their developmental levels, interests, and life goals. This section explains how to identify, adapt, or create resources that foster engagement and promote communication and independence.

Characteristics of Effective Resources

When selecting or creating resources, prioritize materials that are:

- **Age-respectful:** Content should reflect the maturity and interests of middle and high school students, even if it's simplified in complexity. Avoid materials that feel juvenile or patronizing.
- **Functionally relevant:** Resources should address real-life skills, such as navigating the community, managing money, or participating in social interactions.
- **Flexible and adaptable:** Materials that can be tailored to meet individual communication needs (e.g., visual, verbal, tactile) are ideal for life skills students.

- **Engaging and motivating:** Use resources that resonate with the student's interests, such as pop culture, music, sports, or technology.
- **Culturally and linguistically appropriate:** Ensure that resources are inclusive and reflect the backgrounds and experiences of your students.

Recommended Types of Resources

Here are some categories of resources and specific examples to consider.

Visual supports:

- **Visual schedules:** Use apps like Choiceworks or printed templates to help students understand routines and transitions.
- **Picture cards:** Tools like Boardmaker, SmartySymbols, or LessonPix or free resources from sites like Teachers Pay Teachers (TPT) offer visuals for requesting, sequencing, or identifying emotions.
- **Video modeling:** YouTube or other video platforms can provide examples of social interactions, vocational tasks, or daily routines.

Community-based materials:

- **Real-life flyers and menus:** Collect menus, store flyers, or public transportation schedules for activities like ordering food, budgeting, or planning a trip.
- **Maps:** Use printed or digital maps to teach students how to navigate their school, community, or public transportation routes.
- **Functional worksheets:** Create or download resources focused on skills like writing a grocery list, budgeting for a shopping trip, or planning daily schedules.

Digital tools and apps:

- **AAC and communication apps:** Try apps like Proloquo2Go, TouchChat, CoughDrop, PRC-Saltillo, and others for students using AAC devices. There are many available, you just need to find the right one to meet the needs of your student.
- **Interactive learning platforms:** Use tools like Boom Cards for practicing functional communication in a game-like format.
- **Job skills simulations:** Access virtual job training platforms, such as myinterviewpractice.com or job-applications.com, to introduce vocational tasks in an interactive way.

Literacy and reading resources:

- **Simplified texts:** Use platforms like Tar Heel Reader for high-interest, low-complexity reading materials.
- **Functional literacy materials:** Provide resources for reading signs, instructions, or labels, such as mock recipes, road signs, or job applications.
- **Audiobooks and read-alouds:** Use platforms like Epic! or Audible for students who benefit from auditory input. You can also use storylineonline.net, which has storybooks read by celebrities.

Games and hands-on activities:

- **Functional board games:** Try games like Life Skills Bingo or Pay Day, which focus on real-world tasks.
- **Cooking activities:** Use simple recipes for students to practice following directions, measuring, and sequencing.
- **DIY projects:** Create materials like matching cards for emotions, role-playing scripts, or sorting tasks for job-related skills.

Where to Find Resources

Here are some great places to source life skills resources:

- **Teachers Pay Teachers (TPT):** Offers a variety of free and paid resources tailored to life skills and secondary students.
- **SLP and special education blogs:** There are many blogs like mine at speechtimefun.com that can provide resources and suggestions for working with life skills students. Some SLP Instagram accounts I recommend for working with life skills students are @one.on.one.speechtherapy, @bohospeechie, and @abaspeechbyrose. Some SLP blogs I recommend for AAC support are PrAACtical AAC, Emily Diaz, and Rachel Madel. Some suggested special education blogs are SPED Adulting and Full SPED Ahead.
- **Library and community centers:** Local libraries often have free resources like maps, menus, or literacy materials that can be incorporated into therapy.
- **Vocational and life skills programs:** Partner with organizations or schools that focus on vocational training for access to age-appropriate materials.

- **DIY and free tools:**
  - **Canva:** Create custom visuals and worksheets.
  - **Google Slides or Docs:** Design simple templates for schedules, social stories, or lists.
  - **Open-source materials:** Check websites like ReadWorks for free or low-cost accessible texts.

Adapting Existing Materials

Sometimes, resources need to be adjusted to better fit your students' needs. Here are tips for adapting materials:

- **Simplify language:** Use fewer words, clear vocabulary, and concise sentences for easier comprehension.
- **Add visuals:** Pair text with pictures, diagrams, or symbols to support understanding.
- **Provide scaffolds:** Include templates, sentence starters, or step-by-step guides to help students complete tasks independently.
- **Chunk information:** Break down lengthy materials into smaller sections to avoid overwhelming students.
- **Incorporate personal interests:** Modify the content to include familiar or motivating topics, such as favorite foods, hobbies, or preferred activities.

Collaborating with Others to Source Resources

Collaborating with others can be a great way to access materials:

- **Families:** Ask families to share tools or real-life materials from home (e.g., grocery lists, family schedules, or chore charts).
- **Teachers:** Partner with special education teachers to share classroom resources that align with the student's goals.
- **Local businesses:** Connect with local stores, restaurants, or job sites to collect menus, applications, or practice materials for vocational skills.
- **Online communities:** Join social media groups or forums for SLPs and special educators to find and share life skills resources. SLP Elevate comes with a Facebook community where you can ask questions and get support.

Tips for Success

Consider these tips to help your students be successful:

- **Start simple:** Begin with basic resources that are easy for students to understand and use, then gradually increase complexity as their skills develop.
- **Test and adapt:** Not every resource will work for every student. Be flexible and willing to tweak materials to ensure they are effective.
- **Encourage ownership:** Involve students in creating or choosing their own materials to increase motivation and engagement.
- **Track progress:** Use data to determine which resources are most effective and adjust as needed.

By curating and creating the right resources, you can provide engaging, age-appropriate, and functional therapy that helps life skills students achieve greater independence and success in their daily lives.

SAMPLE SPEECH AND LANGUAGE GOALS FOR LIFE SKILLS STUDENTS

Functional communication goal: The student will independently request preferred items or activities in structured and unstructured settings using verbal language, AAC, or gestures, achieving 80 percent accuracy across three consecutive sessions.

Social interaction goal: The student will initiate and respond to greetings, maintain eye contact, and use appropriate conversational turn-taking with peers and adults in structured role-play scenarios, achieving four out of five successful attempts over three sessions.

Vocational communication goal: The student will follow multistep oral or written directions (two or three steps) related to a vocational task (e.g., sorting, assembling, or preparing materials) with 90 percent accuracy in four out of five opportunities.

Self-advocacy goal: The student will appropriately request clarification or assistance when presented with unclear or challenging tasks in academic or vocational settings, using verbal or nonverbal strategies, in 80 percent of observed opportunities over three weeks.

Functional literacy goal: The student will read and comprehend functional texts (e.g., recipes, safety signs, schedules) and answer WH questions or demonstrate comprehension through task completion with 90 percent accuracy in three out of four trials.

Choosing the Right Therapy Setting

One of the most important decisions SLPs face when working with life skills students is determining the most effective therapy setting—push-in or pull-out. Both approaches offer unique benefits and challenges, and the choice depends on the student's individual needs, goals, and the classroom environment. Push-in therapy provides opportunities for students to practice communication in real-life, natural contexts, while pull-out therapy allows for focused, distraction-free skill building. Finding the right balance ensures that therapy is meaningful, impactful, and tailored to help students achieve independence and functional communication.

I had to make this decision once for my life skills students. The classroom was far from my therapy room, the students struggled with transitioning in and out of the room, my room was too small for incorporating sensory needs, and I didn't have time to collaborate with the teacher. I decided to push-in and work with the students individually in the room. This allowed me to have more time with the students since we weren't transitioning to my room, I had access to the materials that they were using in the classroom, and the teacher and paraprofessionals were able to observe what I was doing with the students so that they could ask questions or assist with carry-over. I have pushed into other classrooms in my career where I was working with the whole class. It was designed so that the teacher could participate in carry-over strategies that I was using with the students. However, the teacher was not receptive or cooperative. She did not want to participate and used my session and a prep period for herself. This push-in situation did not work, and I decided to remove it and switch to pull-out with these students instead.

This section discusses how to determine the appropriate setting for your students.

Understanding the Options

Push-in therapy:

- Is provided directly in the student's classroom environment during natural activities.
- Focuses on supporting communication within the context of daily routines, academic tasks, and social interactions.

Pull-out therapy:

- Is conducted in a separate, quiet environment with fewer distractions.
- Allows for targeted, individualized intervention without the complexities of the classroom.

Factors to Consider

Student-specific needs

- **Strengths:** Students with severe distractions or sensory needs may benefit more from pull-out sessions to focus on skills.
- **Current skills:** Students who struggle with generalizing skills may need push-in services to practice in the natural environment.

Therapy goals

- **Functional communication goals:** If the goal is to increase communication during real-world tasks, push-in may offer a more authentic context.
- **Skill-building:** For foundational skills like AAC navigation or articulation drills, pull-out sessions may be more effective initially.

Classroom environment

- **Collaboration:** Push-in works best when the teacher is open to collaboration and there is a structured environment for the SLP to integrate.
- **Activity fit:** For students in highly individualized or sensory-heavy classroom environments, a pull-out model might reduce overstimulation.

Opportunities for generalization

- Skills like greetings, turn-taking, and group participation benefit from push-in therapy for immediate practice in authentic settings.
- Specialized skills may require pull-out first, followed by push-in for application.

Logistical considerations

- **Class size:** Large, chaotic classes may make push-in less effective.
- **SLP schedule:** Balancing the SLP's availability and the timing of meaningful classroom activities is essential.

> **TIP**
>
> Many students benefit from a blended approach, starting with pull-out therapy to develop the skill and moving to push-in therapy to generalize it in the natural context.

NOW WHAT?

You've explored the strategies, challenges, and resources necessary to make an impact when working with middle and high school life skills students. Now, it's time to put these ideas into practice! Reflect on your current approach, think critically about your next steps, and take immediate action to see a difference in your sessions.

Reflect on your students' needs:

- What functional communication skills are your students currently excelling at, and where are they struggling most?
- Are there gaps between the goals in their IEPs and the practical skills they need in daily life? If so, how can you address those gaps?

Evaluate your approach:

- How often do you incorporate real-life scenarios into your sessions? Could this be increased?
- Are you utilizing your students' strengths to build independence and confidence?
- How effectively are you collaborating with families and other professionals? What could be improved?

Assess your resources:

- Do the materials you use feel age-appropriate and engaging for your students?
- Are your resources functional and aligned with real-world tasks your students will encounter?
- What gaps exist in your current toolkit, and where can you find additional support?

Plan for collaboration:

- How often do you communicate with families about their child's progress and how to practice skills at home?
- Have you reached out to general education teachers, special education teachers, or vocational coordinators to ensure consistency across environments?

Set a vision:

- If you could achieve one major milestone with your students in the next three months, what would it be?
- What changes can you make in your daily practices to ensure students see quick wins that build momentum?

Working with middle and high school life skills students is a unique and deeply rewarding opportunity to make a lasting impact. By focusing on functional communication, fostering independence, and building meaningful collaborations, you can empower your students to navigate their daily lives with confidence and purpose. It's not about achieving perfection in every session, and this is coming from a recovering perfectionist. It is about small, consistent steps that lead to meaningful progress. Remember, your creativity, adaptability, and belief in your students' potential are the most valuable tools you bring to the table. As you put these strategies into action, celebrate the growth you see and the connections you foster. You are not just teaching skills, you're helping shape futures, one practical step at a time.

Conclusion

Congratulations! You made it to the end! I am so excited that you made it to the end of this book. You survived my ramblings and crazy therapy ideas! You decided to read to improve your practice or learn more about working with middle and high school speech students. You can use these ideas with your upper elementary students as well. It is my dream that all SLPs working with secondary students realize it doesn't have to be scary, it doesn't have to be impossible, and that working with this age group can be fun and impactful. Turns out, working with teenagers isn't about being cool—it's about being consistent. They don't care if you know the latest TikTok trend; they care that you care.

It is the best feeling knowing that you can be the one person in that student's life who believes in them, that they can trust, that can show them what is possible, and to make their dreams and goals a reality. So often our students go through their school days lacking confidence, aware of their difficulties, and struggling. We get to build their confidence and make learning fun. We have the best job in the world.

IT IS TIME TO DELIVER

Throughout this book, I discussed how to get quick wins for your students so they will work with you, how to incorporate their interests and goals to keep them motivated and bought-in, and how to plan quickly, even with mixed groups. You can take everything you learned in this book to deliver successful lessons to any group and any group size. Don't overthink it.

Here are the key ingredients to a successful lesson with secondary students:

- **Understanding:** You need to always be understanding what goals to work on that are appropriate for your students, not just what is expected of them in the classroom. How are you teaching it to them differently?

- **Compassion:** You need to always be mindful of your students' feelings about coming to speech and their learning and communication difficulties. They may have been getting speech for years and are tired of it. They are embarrassed. They are constantly reminded of their struggles, such as poor grades, being pulled to the back of the room for help, or even struggling with homework.
- **Adaptability:** Always be looking at activities through the lens of how many goals can you address with them. Also, be willing to pivot if things are too easy or too hard. It is okay to change your game plan mid-lesson. This is why I hate when administrators ask SLPs to submit lesson plans. We cannot always stick to a plan!
- **Creativity:** This isn't about crafts but being able to use students' interests and goals to tailor sessions that are relevant to them. It can be as easy as just using your session introduction and conclusion to show them how they can use the skill in their world.

That's it. With these four key ingredients, you can bring magic to each session. It is possible. It doesn't require hours of preparation. It is possible to plan quickly, still be effective, and have more time for you.

TRIAL AND ERROR

This is just a friendly reminder that our profession involves a lot of trial and error. We do not have a roadmap that works for every student. You need to be okay with trying things, learning from mistakes, and pivoting when necessary. Trial and error is like learning to ride a bike on an unfamiliar trail. At first, you might wobble, hit a few bumps, or even fall. The trail might be uneven, with unexpected twists and turns. But each time you get back on, you learn something new. You learn how to balance better, navigate obstacles, and adjust your speed. Over time, you develop the confidence to ride smoothly, even when the path is challenging.

In speech and language therapy, every student is like a new trail. Every student is unique, with their own challenges and surprises. The key is to keep going, learning from the ride, and knowing that every stumble is part of mastering the journey.

Don't be hard on yourself if a student doesn't pick up a skill right away or if you use materials that are too challenging at first. Brush it off. You can make changes for the next session. That is why goals are annual goals. You have a year to figure them out, practice them, and demonstrate mastery.

MY WISH FOR YOU

I hope you now realize what is possible. I hope you find the joy and fun working with this age group. So many teachers are fearful or hesitant to work with older students. Many are not trained how to work with this age group in graduate school, and many are thrown into settings without support, materials, or someone to turn to. You have me. You have tips and ideas from this book that you can always refer to. You have tons of free resources that are available to you at my website at www.speechtimefun.com/book. You now have the tools to know where to start, ways to target goals, and ways to make sessions relevant and fun.

You can also always reach out to me via social media or email at hallie@speechtimefun.com if you have any questions or need further support. Your journey doesn't stop here. It is just the beginning. You will always have me on your bookshelf and someone to turn to for guidance. I remember what it was like not having someone to turn to. It was not easy and was not fun. I often felt inadequate. It is my mission that secondary SLPs never feel like they are at it alone. I don't want SLPs trying to leave this setting because they are not feeling like they are making an impact or able to do the job they were hired to do. You are amazing. Your students are so lucky to have you as their SLP. They still need you at this age, and there is still so much we can do for them.

NOW WHAT?

Let's keep the dialogue going! Join me on social media, share your successes, and inspire others to fall in love with working with secondary students. Together, we can change the narrative. If you found this book helpful, it would mean the world to me if you would share it with friends and colleagues. Post about your reading it on social media and tag me (@speechtimefun). I am on Instagram, Facebook, and TikTok. I can also be found on LinkedIn as Hallie Sherman. I want to see you reading this book and loving it. I want SLPs everywhere to know that this guide is available and that they are not alone when working with secondary students.

Be the best SLP you can be for your students. Make mistakes. Have fun. Laugh at yourself. Laugh with your students. Smile. Be amazing. Be the SLP you went to graduate school to be. Make a difference each day. Do what you love and love what you do.

If you are still in graduate school, my hope is that this book gave you insights on what you can do when you begin working as an SLP with this age group. Maybe consider trying this age group if you haven't considered it before. Having read this book, you are going into the field knowing a lot more than most SLPs! Share this book with your fellow classmates. Help spread the word that this age group can be the best to work with.

There isn't an award for being the last car out of the parking lot, for bringing the most work home, or always feeling like you are running on empty. This job is important and a big part of our lives, but it shouldn't take over. The more you work smarter not harder and use the principles and strategies in this book, the more work-life balance you will see as a result. Remember, you're not just an SLP—you're a mentor, a cheerleader, and sometimes, the only person in a student's corner. Your work matters more than you know. Keep showing up, keep learning, and keep believing in the power of what you do. Because here's the secret: your students believe in you, too. What are you waiting for? Go get them! Go have fun!

Index

A

AAC *see* augmentative and alternative communication

academics
    basics, 17
    and functional goals, 173
    and language impairments, 16
    standards, 20
    struggles, 17

accountability, 104, 106

active participation, 105
    in class discussions, 125

adaptability, 76, 189, 192

adulthood, 21
    transitioning to, 18, 174

advocates, families as, 180, 181

age-appropriate *vs.* age-respectful material,
    129–130

anchor chart, 10, 14, 51

anxiety, 5, 42, 84, 105–106
    handling test, 59
    reduction of, 105
    for secondary students, 49, 105

articulation, 20, 31, 89, 107, 138, 140–144, 151,
    152, 154–157
    feedback, 165
    ideas for secondary students, 159–162
    joke books, 160
    lyrics showdown, 161
    Mad Libs, 160
    movie voiceover challenge, 161
    pop culture debates, 161
    reflection, 165
    social media influencer simulation, 161
    and social skills activities, 167
    100 trial races, 160
    word searches, 160

artificial intelligence, for educators, 128

aspirations, 78
    academic, 80
    tapping into, 80

audiobooks, 183

auditory learners, 44, 54–55

auditory tools, 56

augmentative and alternative communication (AAC)
    and communication apps, 182
    users, 175

availability, 119
    student schedules, 148

B

background knowledge, 12, 128, 214
    lack of, 15
    language activities, 5
    language comprehension, 11

batch planning
    in action, 139–140
    benefits, 137
    implementation, 138–139
    session, 139
    using versatile materials, 140–142

behavior
    challenges, 173
    issues, 105
    off-task, 104
    reinforce positive, 173
    social, 172

Bloom, Benjamin, 26

Bloom's Taxonomy, 26–27, 32

books, 13, 142
    ELA, 43
    vocabulary, 142

Boom Cards, 139, 182

boundary setting, 118–120

buffer time, 120

burnout, 116, 119, 136
    prevention, 119

C

Canva, 184

carrier phrases, 53–54

caseload management, 67, 77, 99, 100, 109
challenge chart
    growth mindset, 96
    scheduling, 125
    vocabulary, 96
chaos management, 104, 112
chunking strategy, teaching strategies, 46, 49–50
classroom
    activities, curriculum, 124
    AI to adapt materials, 128
    discussions, 125
    environment, 187
    fifth and sixth graders challenges, 101
    life skills, 176
    lighting, 59
    noisy, 59
    repetition instruction, 58
    reward system in, 100
    secondary students articulation, 159
    strategies in, 60
CLEAR, 10
cognitive abilities, 173
    graphic organizers, 44
    load, 47
collaboration
    on data tracking, 179
    with families, 178
    plan for, 189
    problem-solving, 150
    strategies for, 179
color-coding
    note-taking strategy, 47–48
    tools for, 48–49
    uses of, 48
comfort contract, rapport, 89–90
commercials and communication skills, 166
CommonLit, 127
communication, 104
    and commercials, 166
    diversity, 171
    fostering relationships, 169
    functional, 169–171, 172
    limited generalization of skills, 172
    to meet basic needs, 169
    multimodal, 172
    self-advocacy, 170
    skills, 17
    SLP's role, 170
    styles, 151
    thorough assessments, 171
    using games, 166–167
    wants and needs, 120
communication skills
    through article, 155–156
    workplace, 176
    YouTube Video, 153
community-based materials, 182
community resources, 175
compassion, 192
confidence, 105, 151, 157, 158
    and independence, 170
    issues, 172
    middle and high school life skills students, 189
    and self-worth, 170
consistency, 70, 137, 143
    and clarity, 118
    and structure, 104
contextualized learning, 69
cooking, 177
    activities, 183
creative competence, 76–77
creativity, 143, 192
    extensions, 165
critical thinking, 10, 17, 124
cueing, teaching routine, 103
curriculum, 6, 19, 41, 87, 123
    benefits of breaking free from, 124–125
    challenges, 125
    classroom, 124
    goal on, 28–29, 34
    grade-level, 131–132
    materials, 132
    materials in speech therapy, 133
    vocational themes, 176

D

D'Amelio, Charli, 93
data collection, 63, 71
    alternatives, 69
    anecdotal logs, 69
    data priorities, 157
    one goal at time per student, 156
    organization, 156
    parent and teacher input, 70
    peer participation, 157
    technology use for efficiency, 157
    tips and tricks, 156–157
data-sharing system, 179
decision-making, 170
dice, 141, 160
digital resources, 136–137, 139
digital tools and apps, 182

Disney, Walt, 92
disorganization, 118
DIY projects, 183, 184
DOGO News, 128
Downey Jr., Robert, 93
dry erase board
    and markers, 141
    vocabulary, 141
dynamic and flexible therapy, 151

E

Edison, Thomas, 92
efficiency, 137, 142–143
    batch-plan for, 121
    technology use for, 157
    and time savings, resources, 142
Eisenhower Matrix, 113–115
employment readiness, 170, 174
engagement, 150, 154
English language arts (ELA) workbooks, 4
Epic! platform, 127, 183
ESL worksheets, 4
executive function, 13
expectations, 10, 99–100, 101–102
    benefits of rules and, 103–106
extracurricular, 60

F

failures
    famous, 91
    stories as inspiration, 93
    successful, 92
    without explanation, repeated, 16
families
    collaboration with, 174, 178, 184
    in strategy selection, 181
favorites and preferences, 78
feedback
    communication, 156
    delivery, 107
    within group, 152
    peer, 70
    types of, 150
    verbal, 154
fixed mindset, 94, 95
flashcards
    color-coded, 48
    with images, vocabulary, 52
    learning process, 137
Fleming, Alexander, 92
flexibility, 127, 137, 151, 180

flexible seating options, 107
flyers, 174, 182
Fry, Art, 92
fun and games, in speech therapy, 84–85
functional communication, 188
    goal, 185
    and independence, 169–171
    skill-building, 187
    therapy goals, 187
functional literacy goal, 185

G

games
    and communication, 166–167
    and hands-on activities, 183
    with open-ended questions, 141
    in speech therapy, 84–85
gamify it, teaching routine, 103
gaming commentary practice, 161, 164, 165
generalization, 150
goal
    academic, 79–81
    annual *vs.* session, 25
    appropriate, 39–42
    bad, 36–39
    collaboration, 34–35
    confident with, 8
    creation, 7
    on curriculum, 28–29
    on curriculum alone, 34
    goal-driven activities, 151
    good, 36–39
    identification, 138
    improvement of, 36–39
    language comprehension, 43
    mistakes, 30
    overly complex, 33
    personal, 79–81
    realistic, 137
    and recommendations, 28
    revisiting, 35–36
    setting attainable, 24–36
    setting unrealistic, 33
    understanding, 191
    using negative language, 35
    vocabulary, 151
Goldilocks Rule, 132
Google Drive, 139
Google Images, 167
Google Slides/Docs, 184
grammar, 15, 31

graphic organizers, 141
    language comprehension and, 44
    teaching strategies with, 45–46
growth mindset, 94, 95
    challenge chart, 96
    model and practice, 96

H

Harry Potter, 93
high-school
    life skills, 181
    speech students, goal setting, 23
hobbies and activities, 76, 78, 82, 96, 117, 184
homework, 14, 58, 59, 156, 192

I

independence, 18, 170, 185, 189
Individualized Education Plans (IEPs), 3, 4
    rubrics/checklists, 70
interaction, 141
    encourage peer, 152
    learning platforms, 182
interests, students, 77–79
    goal-oriented lessons, 81–82
    interest-based lessons, 81
interviewing, 174, 178
    during speech time, 178

J

job, 175, 176
    communication skills, 174
    skills simulations, 182
jokes, 142, 160
Jordan, Michael, 92

K

knowledge
    background, 12, 128, 214
    lack of, 15
    language activities, 5
    language comprehension, 11
    language structures, 13
    literacy, 13

L

language, 152
    activities, 130
    for life skills students, 185
    negative, 35
    simplification, 184
    skills, 124, 125
    structures, 11, 13

language comprehension, 5, 28, 89, 151, 155, 157, 159
    components, 11, 22
    goals, 43
    graphic organizers and, 44
    improvement strategy, 53
    language weaknesses, 16
    literacy concepts, 13
    SLP in, 7
language impairments, 11, 14–21
    older *vs.* younger students, 16–18
learning
    materials, 27
    from mistakes, 192
    multifaceted opportunities, 150
    younger students, 17
lesson planning, 111, 120
library, 99
    and community centers, 183
    digital, 127
life after school, 18
life skills, 169
    students, 185
literacy-based therapy, 3
literacy knowledge, 11, 13–14
local businesses collaboration, 184
lyrics
    articulation showdown, 161
    song, 142
    TikTok scripts, 160

M

maps, 125, 182
Marvel's the Avengers, 93
materials, 145
    batch planning session, 139
    organization of, 138
    overwhelm, 136
    prep process, 137
    quantity of, 137
    standardize and reuse, 136
medication information, 177
menu, 182
    reading and ordering, 177
metacognitive thinking, 50–51
middle-school
    confidence, 189
    life skills, 181
    speech students, goal setting, 23
mindset
    fixed, 95
    growth, 95
    shifts, 149

mistakes
  learning from, 192
  of learning process, 92
  SLPs, 117–118
  vocabulary and goal, 31
mixed-group
  challenge, 148
  fun with, 157–158
  speech groups, 150
  step-by-step process, 151
Monarch Reader, 128
morphemes, 13
movement-based learning, 56
movie voiceover, 161
multifaceted learning opportunities, 150
multigoal strategies, 152
multi-sensory learning, 55–56

N

narrative language, 45
natural reinforcement and competition, 151
NewsELA, 127
note-taking strategies, teaching, 46–47

O

older students
  academic struggles, 17
  confidence, 42
  continued speech services, 20–21
  foundational skills, 32–33
  life after school, 18
  self-advocacy, 18
  SLP role, 21–22
  social and emotional challenges, 17, 17–18
  standardized test, 41–42
  vs. younger, language impairments, 16–18
online communities collaboration, 184
open-source materials, 184
overplanning, 118
overthinking, 64, 117
Oxford Owl, 128

P

participation
  active, 105
  in class discussions, 125
  to extend data opportunities, 157
peer modeling, 150
penicillin, 92
personal insights, 79
phonological awareness, 11, 17, 19
physical workspace, 119

picture cards, 140, 182
planning, 116
  flexible, 151
  lesson, 121
  session, 120, 121
podcast, 161
pop culture and entertainment, 78
post-it notes, 92
predictability, 104, 149
problem-solving, 124
  collaborative, 150
  during difficult task, 51
  skills, 24
professional growth, 69, 75
progress
  difficulty tracking, 144
  monitor and document, 153
prompts, text-based, 141
public transportation, 178
pulling students out, 20
pull-out therapy, 187
push-in therapy, 186–187

Q

Quick Wins Concept, 6

R

rapport, 87, 97
  comfort contract, 89–90
  growth mindset, 94–96
  rapport-building activities, 90–94
Raz-Kids (Learning A-Z), 128
read-aloud, 183
reading
  comprehension, 13, 15, 31, 124
  grade level, 126
  and ordering from menu, 177
reading difficulties, 14
  background knowledge, 15
  social pragmatic deficits, 15–16
  verbal reasoning challenges, 15
  vocabulary deficits, 15
  weak syntax and grammar, 15
reading rope, 11, 18, 21
reading specialist, 4, 5, 9, 10, 19, 27, 126
  role, 19
read out loud, 107
ReadWorks, 127
real photos, 167
real time, 149, 153, 160
real-world, 170, 171
reinforcement, 107

repetitive tasks automation, 139
resources, 174
  adapting, 142–143
  benefits of, 142–143
  categories of, 182
  collaboration, 184
  digital, 136–137
  grade level, 127
  literacy and reading, 183
  multigoal, 138
  overwhelm, 135–136
  risks of, 143–144
  and templates, 136–137
responsibility, 104
reward system, 99
role-playing
  at home, 180
  teaching routine, 103
routines, 99–100, 108
  predictable, 152
  in speech room, 103
  teaching, 103
Rowling, J. K., 93

S

scaffolding, 153, 173
Scarborough, Hollis, 11
scene cards, 140
schedule, SLP, 187
secondary students *see also* older students
  anxiety for, 49, 105
  articulation ideas for, 159–162
  ingredients to successful lesson with, 191
  social media influencer simulation, 162–165
  social skills ideas for, 165–167
self-advocacy, 174
  accommodations, 59–60
  assistance request, 57
  clarification strategies, 57
  confidence to speak up, 57
  goal, 185
  handling test anxiety, 59
  older students, 18
  overwhelm management, 57
  repetition requests, 56
  role-playing scenarios, 58–60
  strategies, 56–58
self-assessments, 69
self-care, 117

self-esteem, 18
self-worth, 170 *see also* confidence
semantics, 13
sensory needs, 59
sentence starters, 53
session planning, 120, 121
Silver, Spencer, 92
60-minute plan strategy, 115–116
SLP Elevate, 128
SMART goals, 31, 34
  reminder, 29–30
social media
  articulation, 161
  influencer simulation, 161, 162
  instructions for students, 163
  reflection post-activity, 163
  sample scripts, 162
social skills, 17, 152
  and articulation, 167–168
  goals, 185
  practice, 150
social stigma, 172
song lyrics, 142
special education blogs, 183
speech services
  continuation of, 20–21
  fun activities during, 177
  IEP, 6
  interview skills during, 178
  and language goals, 145, 150
  for life skills students, 185
  mixed groups, 157
  secondary students, 9
Story sequencing cue cards, 52
Storyworks (Scholastic), 127
stress reduction, 137
students *see also* older students
  engagement, 143
  middle-school (*see* middle-school)
  secondary students (*see* secondary students)
  skills, 187
  strengths, 187
  younger, 16–18
syntax, 13–16, 19, 20, 124, 152

T

tactile tools, 55
Tar Heel Reader, 128
task card game, 144

teachers
    collaboration, 184
    curriculum and, 125
    data collection, 70
    role of, 19
Teachers Pay Teachers (TPT), 139, 183
teaching strategies, 43
    chunking strategy, 49–50
    color-coding note-taking strategy, 47–48
    data collection, 64–65
    with graphic organizers, 45–46
    metacognitive thinking, 50–51
    note-taking strategies, 46–47
    using visual aids, 50
technology in therapy, 59, 121, 157
test scores, 20, 32, 33, 42
text-based prompts, 141
    vocabulary, 141
therapy setting, 186
think-aloud, complex text reading, 51
30-minute sample lesson plans, 153
TikTok, 93
    script practice, 161
time
    efficiency, 150
    and energy, 118
    management, 106, 122
    savings, 142–143
    time is money, 112
topic/theme selection, 107
transportation, public, 178, 182
trial and error, 192
turn-taking, 152
two-way partnership, 180

V

verbal reasoning, 11, 13, 14, 26
    challenges, 15, 21
video modeling, 182
visual aids, 51–52
    using teaching strategies, 50

visual supports, 182
    home use, 180
    teaching routine, 103
vocabulary, 14, 22, 25, 38, 175
    age-appropriate, 17
    books, 142
    building, 48
    challenge chart, 96
    deficits, 15
    definition, 12
    dry erase board, 141
    flashcards with images, 52
    goal-driven activities, 151
    and goal mistakes, 31
    and movement-based learning, 56
    text-based prompts, 141
    tier 2 words, 40
    unfamiliar, 47
    visual representations, 51
vocational themes, 176–181
vocational training, 174
    communication goal, 185
    and life skills programs, 183

W

working hours, 119
work-life balance, 111
worksheets, 182
    ESL, 4
    functional, 182
writing skills, 20, 125
writing utensils, 107
wrong answers quiz, 93

Y

"yet" usage
    jar, 95
    power of, 94–95
younger students, language impairments,
    16–18
YouTube videos, 6, 142, 153